The Complete Guide to Aura Healing: Understanding and Repairing Your Energy Field

PUBLISHED BY : Esha x Shiva

Copyright Page

The Complete Guide to Aura Healing: Understanding and Repairing Your Energy Field

Copyright © [2025] [Esha x Shiva]

All rights reserved. No part of this book may be reproduced, distributed, or transmitted in any form or by any means, including photocopying, recording, or other electronic or mechanical methods, without the prior written permission of the publisher, except in the case of brief quotations embodied in critical reviews and certain other non commercial uses permitted by copyright law.

The content in this book is intended for informational and educational purposes only. The author and publisher make no guarantees about the outcome of following the advice contained herein. Readers are encouraged to consult financial, career, and personal development professionals for guidance specific to their circumstances.

Printed in

All content within this book is the intellectual property of the author. Unauthorized reproduction or distribution is prohibited.

Table of Content

Introduction 4

Chapter 1 - The Nature of Energy Fields..11

Chapter 2 - Understanding Your Aura: The Layers of Energy 18

Chapter 3 - The Chakra System and Your Aura 30

Chapter 4 - Aura Colors and Their Meanings 45

Chapter 5 - Learning to See Auras: Techniques for Beginners 56

Chapter 6 - Beyond Seeing: Sensing and Feeling Auras 69

Chapter 7 - Common Aura Disruptions and Their Causes 79

Chapter 8 - The Physical Manifestation of Aura Problems 89

Chapter 9 - Emotional Healing and Your Aura................................101

Chapter 10 - Cleansing Techniques: Removing Negative Energy..113

Chapter 11 - Repairing Tears and Holes in Your Energy Field 128

Chapter 12 - Crystal Healing for Aura Repair 141

Chapter 13 - Color Therapy and Light Work...................................151

Chapter 14 - Sound and Vibrational Healing for Your Energy Field 161

Chapter 15 - Protective Practices: Shielding Your Aura.................175

Chapter 16 - Aura Healing Through Meditation and Breathwork 189

Chapter 17 - Energy Exchange: Relationships and Your Aura.......204

Chapter 18 - Environmental Influences on Your Energy Field........218

Chapter 19 - Case Studies: Transformational Healing Stories 235

Chapter 20 - Developing Your Personal Aura Healing Practice 249

Conclusion: Embodying the Living Light...260

Introduction

Have you ever felt an inexplicable connection to someone you've just met, or sensed an unseen presence in a seemingly empty room? Perhaps you've experienced a sudden wave of discomfort in certain environments or found yourself inexplicably drained after interacting with particular individuals. These experiences, often dismissed as mere intuition or coincidence, may actually be glimpses into the fascinating world of human energy fields – the invisible yet powerful auras that surround and influence every aspect of our lives.

Welcome to "The Complete Guide to Aura Healing: Understanding and Repairing Your Energy Field," a comprehensive exploration of the intricate and often misunderstood realm of human energy. In this book, we'll embark on a journey to uncover the mysteries of the aura, delving deep into the science and spirituality behind this fundamental aspect of our existence. Whether you're a seasoned energy worker or a curious newcomer, this guide will provide you with the knowledge and tools to not only understand your own energy field but also to harness its power for healing, growth, and personal transformation.

The concept of auras has been present in various cultures and spiritual traditions for thousands of years, from ancient Eastern philosophies to modern Western metaphysical practices. However, it's only in recent decades that science has begun to catch up with what mystics and healers have long known – that we are, at our core, beings of energy. Quantum physics has revealed that everything in the universe, including our physical bodies, is composed of vibrating energy at its most fundamental level. This understanding has opened up new avenues for exploring the nature of consciousness, health, and human potential, all of which are intimately connected to the state of our energy fields.

As the author of this guide, I bring a unique perspective that bridges the gap between ancient wisdom and modern scientific understanding. My journey into the world of aura healing began over two decades ago when I experienced a profound energetic awakening following a near-death experience. This life-changing event not only opened my eyes to the reality of the human energy field but also ignited a passion for understanding and working with this invisible yet tangible aspect of our being. Since then, I've dedicated my life to studying various energy healing modalities, from traditional practices like Reiki and Qi Gong to cutting-edge techniques informed by quantum physics and neuroscience.

What sets this book apart from others on the subject is its holistic and practical approach to aura healing. Rather than focusing solely on esoteric concepts or abstract theories, we'll explore the aura from multiple angles – scientific, spiritual, and experiential. You'll find a wealth of hands-on techniques and exercises that allow you to directly engage with your energy field, as well as in-depth explanations of the underlying principles that make these practices effective. Moreover, we'll examine how aura health intersects with various aspects of life, from physical well-being and emotional balance to relationships and environmental influences.

Throughout this guide, we'll explore several key themes and concepts that are essential to understanding and working with your aura. First, we'll delve into the nature of energy fields themselves, examining both the scientific evidence for their existence and the spiritual perspectives that have shaped our understanding of them.

You'll learn about the different layers of the aura, each with its own unique properties and functions, and how these layers interact to create your complete energetic signature.

Another crucial concept we'll explore is the intimate connection between the chakra system and the aura. The seven major chakras, or energy centers, play a vital role in the health and functioning of your energy field. We'll investigate how blockages or imbalances in these chakras can manifest as disruptions in your aura, and conversely, how working with your aura can help to balance and activate your chakras.

Color interpretation is another fascinating aspect of aura work that we'll cover in depth. The colors that appear in your energy field can provide valuable insights into your emotional state, physical health, and spiritual development. You'll learn how to interpret these colors and their various combinations, as well as how to use color therapy to promote healing and balance in your aura.

Perhaps one of the most exciting themes we'll explore is the development of aura perception skills. Many people believe that the ability to see or sense auras is a rare gift, but in reality, it's a skill that can be learned and cultivated by anyone with patience and practice. We'll provide step-by-step instructions for developing your ability to perceive auras visually, as well as techniques for sensing and feeling energy fields through other means.

Lastly, a significant portion of the book is dedicated to practical healing techniques for addressing common aura disruptions and promoting overall energetic well-being. From cleansing and repair methods to protective practices and daily maintenance routines, you'll gain a comprehensive toolkit for keeping your energy field healthy and vibrant.

This book is designed for a wide range of readers, from those who are entirely new to the concept of auras to experienced energy workers looking to deepen their understanding and expand their practice. If you're curious about the unseen energies that influence your life, seeking ways to improve your physical and emotional well-being, or looking to develop your intuitive and healing abilities, you'll find valuable insights and practical tools within these pages.

For the skeptics and scientifically-minded readers, this guide offers a bridge between the mystical and the empirical, presenting evidence-based explanations alongside traditional wisdom. For those already familiar with energy work, you'll discover new perspectives and advanced techniques to enhance your practice. And for individuals struggling with physical or emotional challenges, the healing methods presented here offer a complementary approach to conventional treatments, addressing the energetic roots of dis-ease and promoting holistic wellness.

By engaging with the material in this book, you'll gain a profound understanding of your own energy field and its impact on every aspect of your life. You'll learn to perceive and interpret auras, giving you deeper insights into yourself and others. The healing techniques you'll master will empower you to address energetic imbalances, release emotional blockages, and promote physical healing from within. Moreover, you'll develop a heightened awareness of the energetic dynamics at play in your relationships and environment, allowing you to create more harmonious and supportive conditions for your overall well-being.

Beyond the personal benefits, the knowledge and skills you'll acquire can have a ripple effect on the world around you. As you learn to manage and elevate your own energy, you'll naturally influence the energy of those around you in positive ways. The protective and boundary-setting techniques you'll learn will help you navigate challenging situations and relationships with greater ease and grace. And for those called to healing work, this guide can serve as a foundation for developing your abilities to assist others in their energetic healing journeys.

As we embark on this exploration of the human energy field, I invite you to approach the material with an open mind and a willingness to experience. The world of auras and energy healing can sometimes seem abstract or intangible, but I assure you that with practice and patience, you'll begin to perceive and work with these energies as naturally as you do with the physical world around you.

Remember that this journey is not just about acquiring knowledge, but about experiencing a profound shift in how you perceive yourself and the world. Each chapter builds upon the last, guiding you through a progressive understanding of aura healing that integrates theory with practice. I encourage you to take your time with the exercises and techniques presented, allowing yourself to fully absorb and integrate each new skill before moving on.

Throughout the book, you'll find case studies and personal anecdotes that illustrate the transformative power of aura healing. These real-life examples serve not only to demonstrate the practical applications of the techniques we'll explore but also to inspire you with the possibilities for your own healing and growth. From individuals who have overcome chronic pain and illness to those who have experienced profound spiritual awakenings, these stories highlight the diverse ways in which aura work can catalyze positive change in one's life.

As we delve into the various methods of aura healing, you'll discover that this practice is not just about addressing problems or fixing what's broken. It's about optimizing your energy field to support your highest potential in all areas of life. Whether you're seeking to enhance your creativity, improve your relationships, boost your professional success, or deepen your spiritual connection, a healthy and balanced aura provides the energetic foundation for realizing your goals and dreams.

One of the most empowering aspects of aura healing is that it puts the tools for well-being directly into your hands. While there's certainly value in working with experienced healers and practitioners, the techniques you'll learn in this book will enable you to take charge of your own energetic health on a daily basis. This self-empowerment is particularly important in today's fast-paced and often stressful world, where our energy fields are constantly bombarded with various influences and demands.

As we progress through the chapters, you'll notice that the concepts and techniques build upon each other, creating a comprehensive system for understanding and working with your aura. We'll start with the basics of energy field awareness and gradually move into more advanced practices. By the end of the book, you'll have a robust toolkit for aura healing that you can adapt and personalize to suit your unique needs and circumstances.

It's worth noting that while this guide is thorough and detailed, the world of energy healing is vast and ever-evolving. The knowledge and techniques presented here provide a solid foundation, but I encourage you to view this book as a starting point for your ongoing exploration of aura healing. As you practice and gain experience, you may find yourself drawn to particular aspects of this work or inspired to explore related modalities. Trust your intuition and allow your journey with energy healing to unfold organically.

Finally, I want to emphasize that working with your aura is a deeply personal and often transformative process. As you begin to clear blockages, heal old wounds, and align your energy field, you may experience shifts in various aspects of your life. Relationships may change, new opportunities may arise, and you may find yourself naturally drawn to lifestyle choices that better support your energetic well-being. Embrace these changes as part of your growth and trust in the wisdom of your own energy field to guide you towards greater balance and fulfillment.

As we stand at the threshold of this journey into the world of aura healing, I invite you to take a moment to set your intention for this exploration. What do you hope to gain from this book? What areas of your life are you seeking to heal or improve? Hold these intentions lightly as we proceed, remaining open to the unexpected insights and transformations that may unfold along the way.

Now, let's turn the page and begin our deep dive into the fascinating realm of human energy fields. Get ready to discover the invisible forces that shape your reality, unlock your innate healing abilities, and embark on a journey of energetic transformation that will touch every aspect of your life. Welcome to "The Complete Guide to Aura Healing" – your roadmap to understanding, repairing, and optimizing your energy field for a life of greater vitality, clarity, and purpose.

Chapter 1 - The Nature of Energy Fields

In the vast tapestry of existence, there's an invisible force that surrounds and permeates everything—a subtle, yet powerful energy that connects us all. This energy, often referred to as the "life force," is the foundation of what we call energy fields. As we embark on this journey to understand and heal our auras, it's crucial to first explore the fundamental nature of these energy fields.

The Unseen Reality

Close your eyes for a moment and imagine a world beyond what your physical senses can perceive. In this realm, everything—from the tiniest atom to the largest celestial body—is pulsating with energy. This isn't just a flight of fancy; it's a perspective shared by both ancient wisdom traditions and modern scientific understanding.

When I first began my exploration into energy fields, I was skeptical. How could something I couldn't see or touch have such a profound impact on our well-being? But as I delved deeper, I realized that we interact with invisible forces every day. Think about how you can feel the warmth of the sun on your skin or the pull of gravity keeping you grounded. These are tangible effects of energy fields we can't directly observe.

The Scientific Perspective

From a scientific standpoint, energy fields are a well-established concept. In physics, we learn about electromagnetic fields, gravitational fields, and quantum fields. These fields pervade space and interact with matter in ways that shape our physical reality.

Electromagnetic fields, for instance, are created by electrically charged particles. Your body's nervous system relies on electrical signals to function, creating its own electromagnetic field. Scientific instruments like electroencephalograms (EEGs) and magnetoencephalograms (MEGs) can detect and measure these bioelectric fields produced by your brain.

Quantum physics takes this understanding even further. At the quantum level, particles can be described as vibrating fields of energy. The famous double-slit experiment demonstrated that particles can behave like waves, suggesting a fundamental interconnectedness in the fabric of reality.

While these scientific concepts might seem far removed from the idea of auras, they provide a framework for understanding how unseen energies can influence the physical world. Just as the earth's magnetic field can guide migrating birds, the subtle energy fields around and within us may have profound effects on our well-being.

The Spiritual Perspective

Turning to spiritual traditions, we find a rich tapestry of beliefs and practices centered around energy fields. In many of these traditions, the concept of a life force energy is central. This energy goes by many names—prana in Hinduism and yoga, qi or chi in Traditional Chinese Medicine, ki in Japanese practices, and mana in Hawaiian spirituality, to name a few.

I remember attending a qi gong class where the instructor asked us to feel the energy between our palms. As I stood there, hands held slightly apart, I was astonished to feel a tangible sensation—like a magnetic pull or a ball of warmth. This experience opened my eyes to the possibility that these ancient practices might be tapping into something very real, even if it's not easily measured by conventional scientific instruments.

In these spiritual frameworks, energy fields are often seen as the bridge between the physical and the spiritual realms. They're thought to carry information, influence our health and emotions, and connect us to the broader universe.

The Holistic View

As we explore energy fields, it's important to adopt a holistic perspective that integrates both scientific and spiritual understandings. While they may use different language and methods, both approaches point to the existence of subtle energies that play a crucial role in our lives.

This holistic view suggests that we are more than just our physical bodies. We are complex energy systems, constantly interacting with the energies around us. Your thoughts, emotions, and physical state all influence your energy field, and in turn, your energy field affects your overall well-being.

The Aura: Your Personal Energy Field

Now, let's bring our focus to the specific energy field that surrounds your body—your aura. Think of your aura as a luminous cocoon of energy that extends beyond your physical form. It's often described as a series of interpenetrating layers, each corresponding to different aspects of your being: physical, emotional, mental, and spiritual.

Your aura is not static; it's a dynamic, ever-changing field that reflects your current state of being. When you're feeling vibrant and healthy, your aura might be described as bright and expansive. During times of stress or illness, it might appear dull or contracted.

Understanding your aura as an extension of your energy system can be transformative. It means recognizing that your well-being isn't just about what's happening within your physical body, but also about the energetic exchanges occurring in and around you.

The Interconnectedness of Energy Fields

One of the most fascinating aspects of energy fields is their interconnectedness. Just as dropping a pebble in a pond creates ripples that extend outward, our energy fields interact with and influence one another.

Have you ever walked into a room and immediately sensed tension, even if nothing was visibly amiss? Or perhaps you've experienced the uplifting effect of being in nature or in the presence of a particularly positive person. These experiences can be understood as interactions between energy fields.

This interconnectedness has profound implications. It suggests that our personal energy fields don't exist in isolation, but are part of a larger energetic ecosystem. The health of your aura affects not only your own well-being but also influences those around you.

The Impact on Well-being

Understanding energy fields isn't just an intellectual exercise—it has practical implications for our health and well-being. Many alternative and complementary healing practices, from acupuncture to Reiki, are based on the concept of working with these subtle energies to promote healing.

From this perspective, many health issues can be seen as disruptions or imbalances in the energy field. These disruptions might manifest as physical symptoms, emotional disturbances, or mental blocks. By addressing these energetic imbalances, we may be able to support the body's natural healing processes.

I've witnessed this principle in action through my work with clients. One woman came to me suffering from chronic fatigue and recurring headaches. Traditional medical treatments had provided little relief. When we began working on balancing her energy field through various techniques, she started to experience significant improvements in her symptoms.

Cultivating Awareness

As we delve deeper into the world of aura healing, one of the most valuable skills you can develop is awareness of energy fields. This doesn't necessarily mean seeing auras (although we'll explore techniques for that later in the book). Rather, it's about tuning into the subtle sensations and influences of energy in and around you.

Start by paying attention to how you feel in different environments or around different people. Notice any shifts in your mood, energy levels, or physical sensations. These can be clues to the energetic interactions taking place.

You might also try a simple exercise: Rub your hands together vigorously for a few seconds, then slowly pull them apart. Can you feel a subtle sensation between your palms? This exercise can help you start perceiving the energy field around your own body.

The Journey Ahead

As we conclude this exploration of the nature of energy fields, I hope you're beginning to appreciate the vast and fascinating world that exists beyond our ordinary perception. Understanding energy fields provides a foundation for the healing practices we'll be exploring throughout this book.

In the chapters that follow, we'll delve deeper into the specific layers of the aura, explore techniques for perceiving and working with energy, and learn powerful methods for healing and balancing your energy field. Remember, this is not just about gaining knowledge—it's about embarking on a transformative journey that can enhance every aspect of your life.

The concept of energy fields invites us to expand our understanding of reality and our place within it. It challenges us to consider that we are more than just physical beings, but complex energy systems intimately connected with the world around us. As we continue our exploration, keep an open mind and heart. The nature of energy fields may challenge some of your existing beliefs, but it also opens up exciting possibilities for growth, healing, and connection.

In our next chapter, we'll take a closer look at the specific layers that make up your aura, providing you with a detailed map of your personal energy field. This understanding will serve as a crucial foundation as we move forward in our journey of aura healing and energy field repair.

Remember, the journey of understanding and working with energy fields is deeply personal. As you read on, pay attention to what resonates with you. Trust your intuition and your own experiences. You are embarking on a path of self-discovery that has the potential to transform not only your understanding of yourself but also your relationship with the world around you.

Chapter 2 - Understanding Your Aura: The Layers of Energy

As we delve deeper into the world of aura healing, it's essential to understand the intricate structure of your energy field. In this chapter, we'll explore the various layers that make up your aura, their unique properties, and how they interact with one another to create your complete energy field. By gaining a comprehensive understanding of these layers, you'll be better equipped to identify and address any imbalances or disruptions in your aura, paving the way for more effective healing practices.

The Multidimensional Nature of Your Aura

When I first began my journey into aura healing, I was fascinated by the concept that our energy fields are not just simple, uniform bubbles of light surrounding our bodies. Instead, I discovered that our auras are complex, multidimensional structures composed of several distinct layers, each with its own unique purpose and characteristics.

Think of your aura as a set of Russian nesting dolls, with each layer encapsulating the ones beneath it. These layers extend outward from your physical body, becoming progressively more subtle and expansive as they move further away. Each layer corresponds to different aspects of your being – physical, emotional, mental, and spiritual – and together, they form a holistic representation of your entire energetic makeup.

The Seven Main Layers of the Aura

While some esoteric traditions recognize more than seven layers, for the purposes of this book, we'll focus on the seven main layers that are most commonly identified and worked with in aura healing practices. As we explore each layer, I encourage you to visualize them surrounding your body, starting from the innermost layer and expanding outward.

1. The Etheric Layer

The etheric layer is the first and innermost layer of your aura, extending about 2-4 inches from your physical body. This layer is closely connected to your physical health and vitality, acting as a blueprint for your physical form. When you look at someone's etheric layer, you might perceive it as a faint, bluish-white glow outlining their body.

In my early days of aura reading, I remember working with a client who had recently undergone surgery. As I observed her etheric layer, I noticed a distinct disruption in the energy flow around the area of her incision. This experience taught me how closely the etheric layer mirrors our physical state and how it can be used as a diagnostic tool for identifying areas of physical distress or imbalance.

The etheric layer is also closely associated with physical sensations and instincts. It's through this layer that you might feel a "gut reaction" to a person or situation before your conscious mind has had time to process the information. Paying attention to these subtle physical cues can be an excellent way to begin developing your aura sensing abilities.

2. The Emotional Layer

Moving outward, we come to the emotional layer, which extends about 1-3 inches beyond the etheric layer. As its name suggests, this layer is closely tied to your feelings and emotions. It's often described as being fluid and colorful, with the colors and patterns shifting in response to your emotional state.

I once worked with a young woman who was going through a difficult breakup. As we began our session, I observed her emotional layer swirling with deep blues and purples, indicating her sadness and emotional pain. As we talked and worked through some healing techniques, I watched in amazement as flashes of bright yellow began to appear, signaling the emergence of hope and optimism.

The emotional layer is where we store our feelings, both current and past. Unresolved emotional issues or traumas can create distortions or blockages in this layer, which can then affect our overall emotional well-being. By working with the emotional layer, we can release trapped emotions and promote greater emotional balance and harmony.

3. The Mental Layer

The third layer of the aura is the mental layer, which extends about 3-8 inches beyond the emotional layer. This layer is associated with your thoughts, beliefs, and intellectual processes. It's often perceived as having a more structured appearance than the emotional layer, sometimes described as resembling a finely woven mesh or net of light.

I recall working with a client who was struggling with negative self-talk and limiting beliefs. As I observed his mental layer, I could see areas where the energy appeared tangled and knotted, reflecting the mental loops and patterns he was stuck in. Through our work together, focusing on reframing his thoughts and beliefs, we were able to gradually smooth out these tangles, leading to greater mental clarity and a more positive outlook.

The mental layer is where our thought forms reside. These are energetic constructs created by our habitual thoughts and beliefs. Positive, empowering thoughts create bright, clear thought forms that enhance our overall energy field. Conversely, negative or limiting thoughts can create dense, dark thought forms that can obstruct the flow of energy through our aura.

4. The Astral Layer

The fourth layer of the aura is the astral layer, also known as the bridge layer. This layer extends about 6-12 inches beyond the mental layer and serves as a connection between the physical and spiritual aspects of our being. The astral layer is often associated with our relationships, both with others and with our higher self.

In my experience, the astral layer often appears as a shimmering, rainbow-like field of energy. It's through this layer that we form energetic connections or "cords" with other people. These cords can be healthy and supportive, like the loving bond between partners or close friends, or they can be draining and unhealthy, as in the case of codependent or toxic relationships.

I once worked with a couple who were having relationship difficulties. As I observed their astral layers, I could see thick, tangled cords connecting them, reflecting the complexity and intensity of their emotional connection. Through our work together, focusing on healing past hurts and improving communication, I watched as these cords became clearer and more harmonious, mirroring the positive changes in their relationship.

The astral layer is also where we often experience psychic phenomena and intuitive insights. It's through this layer that we can access higher states of consciousness and connect with spiritual guidance.

5. The Etheric Template Layer

The fifth layer of the aura is the etheric template layer, which extends about 1.5-2 feet beyond the astral layer. This layer acts as a template or blueprint for the etheric layer, and by extension, for your physical body. It contains the perfect pattern for health and vitality, which the lower layers then manifest to the best of their ability.

When I first learned about the etheric template layer, I was struck by its potential for healing. By working with this layer, we can reinforce the ideal pattern of health, helping to guide the physical body towards its optimal state. This layer is often perceived as having a cobalt blue color and a more structured appearance than the lower layers.

I remember working with a client who was recovering from a long-term illness. As we focused on strengthening and aligning her etheric template layer, I could see the energy becoming more vibrant and structured. Over time, this work seemed to support and accelerate her physical healing process, as if we were providing her body with a clearer blueprint to follow.

The etheric template layer is also associated with sound healing. Practices like using tuning forks or singing bowls can be particularly effective in working with this layer, as the sound vibrations can help to reinforce and strengthen the template of perfect health.

6. The Celestial Layer

The sixth layer of the aura is the celestial layer, also known as the spiritual layer. This layer extends about 2-2.5 feet beyond the etheric template layer and is associated with higher states of consciousness, spiritual ecstasy, and unconditional love. The celestial layer is often perceived as having a shimmering, golden-white light.

Working with the celestial layer can be a profoundly transformative experience. I recall a meditation retreat where I first truly connected with this layer of my own aura. As I deepened my meditation, I felt enveloped in a warm, golden light, and experienced a sense of boundless love and connection to all things. This experience shifted my perspective on life and reinforced my commitment to spiritual growth and service.

The celestial layer is where we access our higher wisdom and spiritual insights. It's through this layer that we can experience states of enlightenment and cosmic consciousness. When this layer is strong and clear, we often feel a sense of peace, joy, and connection to something greater than ourselves.

7. The Ketheric Template Layer

The seventh and outermost layer of the aura is the ketheric template layer, also known as the causal layer. This layer extends about 2.5-3.5 feet beyond the celestial layer and contains the energetic template for all the other layers of the aura. It's often described as a highly structured egg-shaped field of shimmering, iridescent light.

The ketheric template layer is associated with our higher purpose, our soul's journey, and our connection to the divine or universal consciousness. It contains the information of our past lives, our karmic patterns, and our future potential.

Working with this layer can lead to profound spiritual insights and transformations. I remember a powerful healing session where a client was able to access information from her ketheric template layer. She received clear guidance about her life purpose and was able to see how her current challenges were connected to lessons her soul was seeking to learn. This insight brought her a deep sense of peace and purpose, even in the face of difficulties.

The ketheric template layer is also where we can access universal wisdom and cosmic knowledge. By attuning to this layer, we can tap into the akashic records – the energetic imprint of all that has ever occurred in the universe.

The Interaction Between Aura Layers

While we've explored each layer of the aura separately, it's important to understand that these layers don't exist in isolation. They constantly interact with and influence each other, creating a dynamic, ever-changing energy field.

Think of your aura as a symphony, with each layer representing a different instrument. When all the instruments are in tune and playing harmoniously, the result is beautiful music. Similarly, when all your aura layers are balanced and working together, you experience a sense of overall well-being and vitality.

However, just as a single out-of-tune instrument can disrupt an entire orchestra, an imbalance in one layer of your aura can affect the whole. For example, unresolved emotional issues in the emotional layer can create thought patterns in the mental layer, which in turn can manifest as physical symptoms via the etheric layer.

I once worked with a client who was experiencing chronic headaches. As we explored her aura, we discovered a significant disturbance in her emotional layer related to unexpressed anger. This disturbance was creating tension in her mental layer, which was then manifesting as physical pain in her etheric and physical bodies. By addressing the root cause in the emotional layer, we were able to bring relief not just to her emotions, but also to her physical symptoms.

Understanding these interactions can help you approach aura healing in a more holistic way. Instead of just focusing on the layer where symptoms are manifesting, you can trace the issue back to its source, often in a different layer, and address it there for more effective and lasting healing.

Aura Layers and Personal Growth

As you progress on your personal and spiritual growth journey, you may notice changes in your aura layers. Generally, as we evolve and expand our consciousness, our outer aura layers become more developed and refined.

For instance, someone just beginning their spiritual journey might have very active lower layers (etheric, emotional, mental) but less developed upper layers. As they engage in practices like meditation, energy work, and self-reflection, their upper layers may become more active and expanded.

I've observed this in my own journey and in the journeys of many clients. One particular client comes to mind – a businessman who initially came to me for stress relief. In our first session, his lower aura layers were very active but somewhat chaotic, while his upper layers were barely perceptible. As he committed to a regular meditation practice and began to explore his spiritual side, I watched over the course of several months as his upper layers became increasingly vibrant and structured.

This growth doesn't just affect the individual layers, but also how they interact. As the upper layers develop, they can have a harmonizing effect on the lower layers, leading to greater overall balance and well-being.

Perceiving Aura Layers

At this point, you might be wondering how you can perceive these aura layers for yourself. While we'll dive deeper into aura sensing techniques in later chapters, I want to offer a few initial insights here.

First, it's important to understand that perceiving aura layers is a skill that can be developed with practice. Some people are naturally more sensitive to energy and may find it easier to perceive auras visually. Others might initially sense the aura through other means – as a feeling, an intuitive knowing, or even through physical sensations.

When I first started learning to perceive auras, I found it easiest to sense the etheric layer. I would often feel a slight pressure or tingling sensation when I moved my hand close to someone's body, indicating the edge of their etheric field. As I practiced, I began to perceive the emotional and mental layers as colors and patterns in my mind's eye.

One exercise you can try is to sit in a dimly lit room and focus your gaze slightly to the side of a person or object. Without straining, allow your peripheral vision to pick up any colors, lights, or shadows around the person or object. This technique can help you begin to perceive the etheric and emotional layers.

Remember, everyone perceives energy differently, and there's no "right" way to sense aura layers. Trust your intuition and be patient with yourself as you develop this skill.

The Aura Layers and Chakra System

Before we conclude this chapter, it's important to touch on the relationship between the aura layers and the chakra system, which we'll explore in more depth in the next chapter. The chakras, or energy centers in the body, are closely connected to the layers of the aura.

Each chakra is associated with specific aura layers and influences the energy in those layers. For example, the root chakra is closely tied to the etheric layer, while the crown chakra is associated with the higher spiritual layers.

Understanding this connection can provide valuable insights when working with your aura. Blockages or imbalances in a particular chakra often manifest as disturbances in the corresponding aura layers. Conversely, by working with specific aura layers, we can influence and balance the associated chakras.

I recall working with a client who was experiencing creative blocks. As we examined her aura, I noticed a stagnant energy in her sacral chakra area, which was reflected in her emotional and mental aura layers. By using techniques to stimulate and balance her sacral chakra, we were able to create movement and flow in these aura layers, which helped to unblock her creative energy.

This interplay between the chakras and aura layers highlights the holistic nature of energy healing. By understanding and working with both systems, we can create more comprehensive and effective healing strategies.

Conclusion: Your Unique Energy Signature

As we conclude this exploration of aura layers, I want to emphasize that your aura is as unique as your fingerprint. The particular blend of colors, patterns, and energies in your aura layers creates your individual energy signature.

This uniqueness is something to be celebrated. Just as we each have our own strengths, challenges, and life experiences, our auras reflect our individual journeys and growth. There's no "perfect" aura – what matters is that your energy field is balanced, vibrant, and supportive of your overall well-being.

Understanding the layers of your aura is a powerful step in your healing journey. It provides a framework for identifying areas of imbalance or disruption and offers insights into how different aspects of your being – physical, emotional, mental, and spiritual – are interconnected.

As we move forward in this book, we'll build on this foundation, exploring how to work with your aura layers to promote healing, growth, and spiritual development. In the next chapter, we'll delve into the chakra system and its relationship to your aura, further expanding your understanding of your energetic anatomy.

Remember, the journey of aura healing is a deeply personal one. As you continue to learn and practice, you'll develop your own unique relationship with your energy field. Trust your intuition, be patient with yourself, and remain open to the wisdom and guidance that your aura can provide.

Chapter 3 - The Chakra System and Your Aura

As we delve deeper into the intricate world of energy fields and aura healing, it's crucial to understand the profound connection between your chakras and your aura. These two energetic systems are inextricably linked, working in harmony to maintain your overall well-being. In this chapter, we'll explore how the seven major chakras interact with your aura, and how blockages in these energy centers can significantly impact the health and appearance of your energy field.

The Chakra System: An Overview

Before we dive into the relationship between chakras and your aura, let's take a moment to understand what chakras are and why they're so important. The word "chakra" comes from Sanskrit and means "wheel" or "disk." In the context of energy healing, chakras are spinning vortexes of energy located along the spine, from the base to the crown of your head.

Think of chakras as energy distribution centers in your body. They receive, process, and distribute life force energy throughout your physical and energetic systems. Each chakra is associated with specific physical, emotional, and spiritual aspects of your being. When these energy centers are open and balanced, energy flows freely, promoting health and vitality. However, when chakras become blocked or imbalanced, it can lead to various physical, emotional, and spiritual issues.

As I've worked with countless clients over the years, I've seen firsthand how chakra imbalances can manifest in their lives. One client, Sarah, came to me complaining of chronic fatigue and a lack of motivation. Upon examining her energy field, I noticed that her solar plexus chakra – associated with personal power and self-esteem – was severely underactive. As we worked to balance this chakra, Sarah reported feeling more energized and confident in her daily life.

The Seven Major Chakras and Their Influence on Your Aura

Now that we have a basic understanding of chakras, let's explore each of the seven major chakras and how they interact with your aura. Remember, your aura is a multi-layered energy field that surrounds and interpenetrates your physical body. The state of your chakras directly affects the health and vibrancy of your aura.

Root Chakra (Muladhara)

Located at the base of your spine, the root chakra is associated with feelings of safety, security, and grounding. When this chakra is balanced, you feel stable and connected to the earth. In your aura, a healthy root chakra often manifests as a strong, vibrant red energy at the base of your energy field.

I once worked with a client, John, who had recently lost his job and was struggling with feelings of instability. His aura appeared weak and fragmented near the base, indicating an imbalanced root chakra. Through grounding exercises and visualization techniques, we were able to strengthen his root chakra. As a result, John's aura became more stable and vibrant, and he reported feeling more secure in his daily life.

When the root chakra is blocked or underactive, you might experience:

- Feelings of insecurity or fear
- Financial struggles
- Difficulty manifesting your desires
- A weak or fragmented aura, especially near the base

Sacral Chakra (Svadhisthana)

The sacral chakra, located just below your navel, governs creativity, sexuality, and emotional well-being. A balanced sacral chakra allows for the free flow of emotions and creative energy. In the aura, this often appears as a vibrant orange glow in the lower abdomen area.

I remember working with an artist, Maria, who was experiencing a creative block. Upon examining her aura, I noticed a dull, stagnant energy around her sacral area. Through chakra balancing techniques and creative visualization exercises, we were able to revitalize her sacral chakra. As a result, Maria's aura began to pulse with vibrant orange energy, and she found herself overflowing with new creative ideas.

When the sacral chakra is imbalanced, you might notice:

- Emotional instability
- Creative blocks

- Sexual dysfunction

- A dull or muddy orange color in your aura

Solar Plexus Chakra (Manipura)

The solar plexus chakra, located in the upper abdomen, is associated with personal power, self-esteem, and confidence. When this chakra is balanced, you feel empowered and in control of your life. In the aura, a healthy solar plexus chakra often manifests as a bright yellow energy radiating from the core of your being.

I once worked with a client, David, who was struggling with self-doubt and a lack of confidence in his professional life. His aura appeared dim and constricted around the solar plexus area. Through affirmations and power poses, we were able to activate and balance his solar plexus chakra. As a result, David's aura expanded and brightened, and he reported feeling more confident and assertive in his work environment.

Imbalances in the solar plexus chakra can lead to:

- Low self-esteem

- Lack of motivation

- Digestive issues

- A weak or constricted yellow energy in your aura

-

Heart Chakra (Anahata)

The heart chakra, located in the center of the chest, is the bridge between the lower and upper chakras. It governs love, compassion, and connection. A balanced heart chakra allows for the free flow of love and empathy. In the aura, this often appears as a beautiful green or pink glow emanating from the chest area.

I remember working with a client, Emily, who had recently gone through a difficult breakup and was struggling to open her heart again. Her aura appeared constricted and dull around the heart area. Through heart-opening meditations and forgiveness exercises, we were able to heal and balance her heart chakra. As a result, Emily's aura began to radiate with a soft, pink light, and she reported feeling more open to love and connection in her life.

When the heart chakra is blocked, you might experience:

- Difficulty giving or receiving love

- Feelings of isolation or loneliness

- Holding grudges

- A constricted or dull green/pink energy in your aura

Throat Chakra (Vishuddha)

The throat chakra, located in the throat area, is associated with communication, self-expression, and speaking your truth. When this chakra is balanced, you can express yourself clearly and authentically. In the aura, a healthy throat chakra often manifests as a clear blue energy around the neck and shoulder area.

I once worked with a public speaker, Mark, who was experiencing severe stage fright. Upon examining his aura, I noticed a blocked and constricted energy around his throat area. Through vocal exercises and affirmations, we were able to open and balance his throat chakra. As a result, Mark's aura began to pulse with a vibrant blue light, and he found himself speaking with more confidence and clarity.

Imbalances in the throat chakra can lead to:

- Difficulty expressing yourself

- Fear of public speaking

- Thyroid issues

- A weak or muddy blue color in your aura

Third Eye Chakra (Ajna)

The third eye chakra, located between the eyebrows, governs intuition, insight, and spiritual awareness. When this chakra is balanced, you have a clear vision of your life path and can easily tap into your intuition. In the aura, a healthy third eye chakra often appears as a bright indigo light radiating from the forehead area.

I remember working with a client, Lisa, who was feeling lost and unsure about her life direction. Her aura appeared dim and fragmented around the third eye area. Through meditation and visualization exercises, we were able to activate and balance her third eye chakra. As a result, Lisa's aura began to glow with a brilliant indigo light, and she reported experiencing increased clarity and intuitive insights in her daily life.

When the third eye chakra is blocked, you might experience:

- Lack of direction or purpose

- Difficulty trusting your intuition

- Headaches or eye problems

- A weak or muddy indigo color in your aura

Crown Chakra (Sahasrara)

The crown chakra, located at the top of the head, is associated with spiritual connection, higher consciousness, and enlightenment. When this chakra is balanced, you feel a deep sense of connection to the universe and your higher self. In the aura, a healthy crown chakra often manifests as a radiant violet or white light emanating from the top of the head.

I once worked with a spiritual seeker, Anna, who was struggling to deepen her meditation practice. Upon examining her aura, I noticed a dim and closed energy around her crown area. Through specific meditation techniques and energy work, we were able to open and balance her crown chakra. As a result, Anna's aura began to shine with a brilliant violet light, and she reported experiencing profound spiritual insights and a deeper connection to her higher self.

Imbalances in the crown chakra can lead to:

- Feelings of spiritual disconnection
- Cynicism or lack of faith
- Cognitive issues
- A weak or absent violet/white energy at the top of your aura

How Chakra Blockages Affect Your Aura

Now that we've explored each of the seven major chakras and their relationship to your aura, it's important to understand how blockages in these energy centers can impact your overall energy field. Chakra blockages occur when energy becomes stagnant or imbalanced within a particular chakra. This can be due to various factors, including:

1. Emotional trauma
2. Negative thought patterns
3. Physical illness
4. Unhealthy lifestyle choices
5. Environmental stressors

When a chakra becomes blocked, it affects not only the specific area associated with that chakra but also the flow of energy throughout your entire system. This disruption in energy flow can manifest in your aura in several ways:

Aura Discoloration

Chakra blockages often result in changes to the color and vibrancy of your aura. For example, if your heart chakra is blocked, you might notice that the green or pink energy typically associated with this area becomes dull, muddy, or even absent in your aura. This discoloration can extend beyond the immediate area of the blocked chakra, affecting the overall appearance of your energy field.

Aura Constriction

When chakras are blocked, your aura may appear constricted or compressed in certain areas. This constriction can limit the flow of vital life force energy throughout your system, leading to feelings of stagnation or being "stuck" in various aspects of your life.

Aura Fragmentation

Severe chakra blockages can cause your aura to appear fragmented or "torn." These breaks in your energy field can leave you vulnerable to negative energies and may manifest as feelings of disconnection or vulnerability in your daily life.

Aura Depletion

Chronic chakra imbalances can lead to overall depletion of your aura. This might appear as a general dimming or weakening of your entire energy field, often accompanied by feelings of fatigue, low motivation, or a lack of vitality.

Techniques for Balancing Chakras and Healing Your Aura

Understanding the connection between your chakras and your aura is the first step towards holistic energy healing. By working to balance and align your chakras, you can directly impact the health and vibrancy of your aura. Here are some effective techniques that I've used with clients over the years to balance chakras and heal the aura:

Meditation and Visualization

Guided meditations focused on each chakra can be incredibly powerful for balancing your energy centers and, by extension, your aura. Try visualizing each chakra as a spinning wheel of light, seeing it clear of any blockages and radiating with vibrant color. As you do this, imagine your aura expanding and glowing with renewed vitality.

Color Therapy

Using colors associated with each chakra can help to stimulate and balance these energy centers. This can be done through visualization, wearing specific colors, or surrounding yourself with objects of particular hues. As your chakras respond to these color vibrations, you may notice positive changes in your aura's appearance and energy.

Sound Healing

Each chakra resonates with specific sound frequencies. Using singing bowls, tuning forks, or even vocalizing certain tones can help to clear and balance your chakras. As the sound vibrations work on your energy centers, you may feel a corresponding shift in your aura's energy.

Crystal Healing

Certain crystals are associated with specific chakras and can be used to balance and activate these energy centers. For example, placing a piece of rose quartz on your heart chakra during meditation can help to open and heal this energy center, potentially resulting in a more vibrant and expansive aura.

Yoga and Physical Movement

Certain yoga poses and movements are designed to stimulate and balance specific chakras. Regular practice of these poses can help to keep your energy centers open and aligned, contributing to a healthy and vibrant aura.

Energy Healing Techniques

Modalities such as Reiki, acupuncture, and other energy healing techniques can be highly effective in balancing chakras and healing the aura. These practices work directly with your energy system to clear blockages and promote the free flow of life force energy.

The Ripple Effect: How Healing One Chakra Can Impact Your Entire Aura

It's important to remember that while each chakra is associated with specific attributes and areas of your life, they don't operate in isolation. The chakra system is interconnected, and healing or balancing one chakra can have a ripple effect throughout your entire energy system.

For example, I once worked with a client, Rachel, who was experiencing severe anxiety and insomnia. Upon examining her energy field, I noticed that her root chakra was severely underactive, causing her aura to appear weak and fragmented near the base. However, this imbalance wasn't isolated to her root chakra. The lack of grounding energy was affecting her entire system, causing her heart chakra to overcompensate (appearing as an overly bright, almost frantic energy in her aura) and her third eye chakra to become blocked (manifesting as a dull, cloudy indigo in her energy field).

We focused our healing work primarily on balancing Rachel's root chakra through grounding exercises and energy work. As her root chakra began to strengthen and balance, we observed fascinating changes in her entire aura. The fragmentation near the base began to heal, her heart chakra's energy softened to a more stable and nurturing vibration, and her third eye chakra began to clear, allowing for greater clarity and intuition.

This example illustrates how working with one chakra can initiate a healing process that extends throughout your entire energy system. It's a beautiful reminder of the interconnectedness of our being and the power of holistic healing approaches.

Developing Chakra Awareness for Aura Health

As you continue on your journey of energy healing, developing a keen awareness of your chakras can be incredibly beneficial for maintaining the health of your aura. Here are some practices you can incorporate into your daily life to cultivate this awareness:

1. Daily Chakra Check-ins: Take a few moments each day to tune into each of your chakras. Notice any sensations, colors, or intuitive impressions you receive. Over time, you'll develop a baseline understanding of how your chakras typically feel when balanced.

2. Aura Scanning: Practice scanning your own aura, paying attention to how the energy feels around each chakra area. You might notice variations in temperature, tingling sensations, or visual impressions of color and light.

3. Journaling: Keep a journal of your chakra and aura observations. This can help you identify patterns and track your progress over time.

4. Mindful Living: Begin to notice how different life experiences affect your chakras and aura. For example, you might observe how certain interactions leave you feeling energized or depleted, and which chakras seem to be most affected.

5. Regular Energy Maintenance: Incorporate chakra balancing techniques into your regular self-care routine. This proactive approach can help prevent major blockages from forming and keep your aura vibrant and strong.

Conclusion: The Dance of Chakras and Aura

As we conclude this chapter, I hope you've gained a deeper understanding of the intricate relationship between your chakras and your aura. These two aspects of your energy anatomy are in constant communication, each influencing and reflecting the state of the other.

By nurturing the health of your chakras, you directly contribute to the vitality and resilience of your aura. And as your aura grows stronger and more vibrant, it creates a supportive energetic environment for your chakras to function optimally. It's a beautiful, symbiotic relationship that forms the foundation of your energetic well-being.

Remember, the journey of chakra balancing and aura healing is ongoing. It's not about achieving a perfect state and maintaining it indefinitely, but rather about developing a deep, intuitive relationship with your energy system. By staying attuned to the needs of your chakras and responding with appropriate care and attention, you create the conditions for a radiant, healthy aura that supports you in all aspects of your life.

As we move forward in this book, we'll explore more specific techniques for working with your aura, building upon the foundational understanding we've established here. The connection between your chakras and your aura will continue to be a central theme, informing our approach to energy healing and personal transformation.

In the next chapter, we'll delve into the fascinating world of aura colors and their meanings, providing you with tools to interpret the visual aspects of your energy field. This knowledge will further enhance your ability to understand and work with your chakras and aura as an integrated system. So, take a moment to reflect on what you've learned here, and prepare to expand your understanding even further as we continue our exploration of aura healing.

Esha x Shiva

Chapter 4 - Aura Colors and Their Meanings

As we delve deeper into the fascinating world of auras, we come to one of the most intriguing aspects of energy fields: their colors. The vibrant hues that emanate from our bodies are not just beautiful to behold; they are rich with meaning and insight into our emotional, physical, and spiritual states. In this chapter, we'll explore the rainbow of aura colors and what they can tell us about ourselves and others.

The Spectrum of Aura Colors

When you first begin to perceive auras, you might be overwhelmed by the array of colors you encounter. From soft pastels to vivid neons, each shade carries its own significance. As we explore these colors together, remember that auras are dynamic and ever-changing. The colors you see today may shift tomorrow, reflecting the constant ebb and flow of your energy.

Let's start with the basics. The primary colors of the aura spectrum are red, blue, and yellow. These foundational hues form the basis for all other colors you might encounter in an energy field. As we go through each color, I'll share with you not only its general meaning but also how variations in shade and intensity can alter its interpretation.

Red: The Color of Vitality and Passion

Red is often the first color many people learn to see in auras. It's bold, unmistakable, and carries powerful energy. When you see red in an aura, you're witnessing the life force in its most raw and potent form.

A bright, clear red indicates a person who is energetic, passionate, and full of zest for life. These individuals often have a strong connection to their physical bodies and may excel in sports or physical activities. They're the go-getters, the ones who charge ahead with enthusiasm and aren't afraid to take risks.

However, like all aura colors, red has its nuances. A deep, burgundy red might suggest a person who is grounded and has a strong will. They're often practical and focused on material success. On the other hand, a murky or muddy red can indicate anger, aggression, or unresolved emotional issues.

I once worked with a client named Sarah who came to me feeling stuck in her career. When I looked at her aura, I saw flashes of bright red mixed with muddy patches. This told me that while she had the passion and drive to succeed, something was holding her back. As we worked together to clear the muddiness in her aura, Sarah found the courage to pursue her true calling as an artist, and her aura began to glow with a clear, vibrant red.

Blue: The Hue of Communication and Calm

Blue in an aura often relates to communication, self-expression, and the throat chakra. It's a color that speaks of tranquility, truth, and wisdom. When you see a clear, sky blue in someone's aura, you're likely dealing with an individual who is honest, has a gift for communication, and possesses a calm, soothing presence.

Deeper shades of blue, like royal or navy, often indicate a person with strong intuitive abilities. These individuals may be natural counselors or teachers, with a depth of wisdom that others are drawn to. They often have a sense of inner peace and a strong spiritual connection.

Lighter shades of blue, such as pale blue or turquoise, can suggest a creative and expressive nature. These people often have a gift for articulating complex ideas in simple terms and may excel in fields like writing, public speaking, or the arts.

However, if the blue appears cloudy or gray-tinged, it might indicate difficulties in self-expression or a fear of speaking one's truth. I remember working with a young man named Michael who had a predominantly blue aura, but it was murky and dull. Through our sessions, we discovered that he had been suppressing his true feelings about his career to please his parents. As he learned to express himself authentically, his aura blue brightened dramatically, and he found himself much happier and more fulfilled.

Yellow: The Sunshine of the Aura

Yellow is the color of intellect, mental clarity, and joy. When you see a bright, clear yellow in someone's aura, you're likely dealing with an individual who has a quick mind, enjoys learning, and approaches life with optimism and cheerfulness.

Pale yellow often indicates emerging psychic abilities or spiritual awakening. It's like the first rays of dawn, suggesting new insights and understanding are on the horizon. Golden yellow, on the other hand, speaks of wisdom gained through experience and a strong sense of self-worth.

But yellow, like all colors, has its shadow side. A muddy or brownish yellow can indicate overthinking, mental stress, or difficulty in making decisions. It might suggest that the person is caught in analysis paralysis or struggling with self-doubt.

I once worked with a brilliant scientist named Elena who came to me feeling burned out and questioning her career choice. Her aura was a mix of bright yellow and murky brown-yellow. The bright yellow showed her natural intelligence and love of learning, but the murky areas revealed her mental exhaustion and self-doubt. As we worked on balancing her energy and reconnecting with her passion for science, the muddy areas cleared, leaving her aura a radiant, sunny yellow.

Green: The Heart of the Matter

Green is the color most associated with the heart chakra, representing love, healing, and growth. A clear, emerald green in the aura suggests a person who is compassionate, nurturing, and in harmony with nature. These individuals often have a healing touch and may be drawn to professions in healthcare or environmental work.

Lighter shades of green, like mint or sage, can indicate a period of growth and change. It's the color of new beginnings, fresh starts, and budding potential. Dark, forest green often suggests a connection to the natural world and may be seen in the auras of those who feel most at home in the wilderness.

However, a murky or olive green can indicate jealousy, resentment, or feeling 'stuck' in one's personal growth. I remember a client named Thomas who came to me struggling with feelings of jealousy in his relationship. His aura was a swirling mix of muddy green and red. As we worked through his insecurities and helped him cultivate self-love, the green in his aura cleared to a beautiful, healing emerald.

Purple: The Color of Spiritual Connection

Purple in an aura is often associated with spiritual awareness, psychic abilities, and a connection to higher realms of consciousness. A clear, vibrant purple suggests someone who is intuitive, visionary, and in touch with their spiritual nature.

Lighter shades of purple, like lavender, can indicate a gentle, sensitive nature and budding psychic abilities. Deeper shades, like indigo or violet, often appear in the auras of spiritual teachers, healers, and those with highly developed intuitive gifts.

However, if the purple appears cloudy or muddy, it might suggest spiritual confusion or misuse of psychic abilities. I once worked with a woman named Amelia who was exploring her psychic gifts but felt overwhelmed and uncertain. Her aura was a swirling mix of muddy purple and gray. As we worked together to ground her energy and develop a structured approach to her spiritual practice, her aura purple cleared and brightened, reflecting her growing confidence and clarity.

Orange: The Color of Creativity and Vitality

Orange in an aura is a joyful, creative color. It speaks of enthusiasm, adventurousness, and a zest for life. When you see a clear, bright orange, you're likely dealing with someone who is sociable, confident, and full of creative energy.

Softer shades of orange, like peach, can indicate a gentle, nurturing energy and a gift for working with others. Deeper, burnished orange often appears in the auras of those who have overcome significant challenges and gained wisdom and strength in the process.

However, a muddy or brownish orange can suggest addictive tendencies or an imbalance in one's creative expression. I remember working with an artist named Jack who was struggling with creative block. His aura was a dull, muddy orange. As we worked to clear his creative channels and address his self-doubt, his aura orange brightened to a vibrant, glowing hue, and his artistic inspiration returned in full force.

Pink: The Hue of Love and Compassion

Pink in an aura is often associated with love, compassion, and nurturing energy. A soft, rose pink suggests a gentle, loving nature and a capacity for deep empathy. Brighter shades of pink can indicate romantic love or a period of opening one's heart to new connections.

Hot pink or magenta in an aura often appears in individuals who have a passionate approach to life and love. These people tend to throw themselves wholeheartedly into their relationships and pursuits.

However, if the pink appears faded or grayish, it might indicate disappointment in love or a closing off of one's heart due to past hurts. I once worked with a woman named Olivia who had recently gone through a difficult breakup. Her aura was a pale, washed-out pink. As we worked on healing her heart and rebuilding her self-love, the pink in her aura gradually deepened and brightened, reflecting her growing capacity to love and be loved.

White: The Color of Purity and Protection

White in an aura is often seen as a protective or purifying color. It can indicate a period of cleansing or a need for purification. Bright, clear white suggests spiritual purity and a high level of consciousness.

Opaque white often appears as a protective layer in the auras of empaths or highly sensitive individuals. It acts as a shield, helping to filter out overwhelming external energies.

However, if the white appears dingy or gray-tinged, it might suggest feelings of isolation or disconnection from one's spiritual nature. I remember working with a highly sensitive client named Liam who felt overwhelmed by the energy of others. His aura had a thick layer of dingy white. As we worked on strengthening his energetic boundaries and connecting with his inner guidance, the white in his aura became clearer and more radiant, providing him with natural protection without cutting him off from others.

Black: Absence or Protection?

Black in an aura is often misunderstood. While it can indicate areas of blocked or absent energy, it can also be a color of protection and grounding. Dense black spots in an aura might suggest areas where energy is stuck or where there's unresolved trauma or fear.

However, a shimmering black, especially around the edges of the aura, can be a sign of protection. Some highly spiritual individuals may have a black aura as a way of shielding their intense energy and preventing overwhelm.

I once worked with a spiritual teacher named Maya whose aura was a deep, shimmering black. Far from being negative, this black was like the night sky - vast, mysterious, and full of hidden depth. It served to contain her immense spiritual energy and allowed her to move through the world without overwhelming others.

The Interplay of Colors

As we've explored the meanings of individual colors, it's important to remember that auras are rarely just one color. Most people have a combination of colors in their aura, and these colors interact and influence each other.

For example, you might see someone with a predominantly blue aura with flashes of red. This could indicate a person who is generally calm and communicative (blue) but also has passion and drive (red) that comes out in certain situations.

Or you might encounter someone with a swirling mix of green and purple, suggesting a person who combines a loving, healing nature (green) with spiritual awareness and intuition (purple).

The way colors blend and interact in an aura can provide deep insights into a person's nature and current state. A harmonious blend of colors often indicates balance and well-being, while sharp contrasts or muddy mixtures might suggest internal conflicts or areas of growth.

Patterns and Shapes in Auras

In addition to colors, auras can display various patterns and shapes, each with its own significance. Spots or flecks of color might indicate temporary influences or emerging traits. Stripes or bands of color could suggest strong, established characteristics or current life themes.

Some people might have swirling patterns in their aura, indicating a period of change or transformation. Others might have a more structured, layered aura, suggesting a well-organized and balanced personality.

I remember working with a client named Sophia who was going through a major life transition. Her aura was a swirling mix of colors, with no clear boundaries between them. As she worked through her changes and found her new direction, her aura began to settle into more distinct layers, reflecting her growing clarity and stability.

The Dynamic Nature of Auras

As we conclude our exploration of aura colors, it's crucial to remember that auras are not static. They change constantly, reflecting our thoughts, emotions, physical health, and spiritual state. The colors you see in your aura or someone else's are a snapshot of the present moment, not a permanent label.

This dynamic nature of auras is what makes them such a powerful tool for self-awareness and growth. By learning to perceive and interpret the colors of your own aura, you gain real-time feedback on your emotional and energetic state. This awareness can help you make conscious choices to shift your energy, address imbalances, and cultivate the qualities you wish to embody.

For instance, if you notice your aura becoming muddy or dull, it might be a sign that you need to take time for self-care or address some unresolved emotions. If you see bright, clear colors emerging, it could be an indication that you're on the right path and your energy is flowing freely.

Developing Your Color Perception

As you continue your journey into aura reading, you'll likely find that your perception of colors becomes more nuanced. You might start to distinguish between different shades of the same color or notice subtle color combinations you hadn't seen before.

This growing sensitivity is a natural part of developing your aura reading skills. Trust your intuition as you interpret what you see. While the general meanings we've discussed in this chapter provide a good foundation, your personal experiences and insights will add depth and nuance to your understanding of aura colors.

Remember, the goal of understanding aura colors isn't to judge or categorize people. Instead, it's to gain insight, foster compassion, and support healing and growth - both for yourself and others.

As we move forward in our exploration of aura healing, we'll build on this understanding of colors to learn practical techniques for cleansing, repairing, and strengthening the aura. The colors you perceive will serve as a guide, helping you identify areas that need attention and showing you the results of your healing work.

In our next chapter, we'll explore techniques for developing your ability to see auras. Whether you're just starting out or looking to refine your skills, you'll find practical exercises to enhance your perception and deepen your understanding of the colorful world of auras.

Chapter 5 - Learning to See Auras: Techniques for Beginners

As we embark on this journey to perceive the unseen, I want you to know that you're about to unlock a remarkable ability that has been dormant within you. Seeing auras isn't a gift reserved for a select few; it's a skill that anyone can develop with patience, practice, and the right guidance. In this chapter, I'll walk you through the process of learning to see auras, sharing techniques that have helped countless beginners, including myself when I first started on this path.

Understanding What We're Looking For

Before we dive into the techniques, it's crucial to understand what exactly we're trying to see. An aura is an electromagnetic field that surrounds all living things, including humans, animals, and even plants. This energy field is often described as a luminous body of light that extends beyond the physical form. When we talk about "seeing" auras, we're really talking about perceiving this energy field with our eyes or our mind's eye.

Auras can appear in various colors, shapes, and intensities. Some people describe them as a hazy glow, while others see distinct layers or patterns. As a beginner, you might start by perceiving a faint, colorless shimmer around objects or people. This is perfectly normal and is an excellent starting point for developing your ability.

Creating the Right Environment

The environment plays a crucial role in your ability to see auras, especially when you're just starting out. I remember when I first began practicing, I would get frustrated trying to see auras in a busy coffee shop or a brightly lit room. It wasn't until I created a dedicated space at home that I started making real progress.

To create an optimal environment for aura viewing, choose a quiet, dimly lit room. Soft, natural light is ideal, so if you can practice near a window on an overcast day, that's perfect. Avoid harsh artificial lighting or complete darkness. The goal is to have just enough light to see clearly without straining your eyes.

Ensure the background behind your subject (whether it's a person, plant, or object) is plain and neutral. A white or light-colored wall works well. Remove any distracting elements from your field of vision. This will help you focus solely on the energy field you're trying to perceive.

Preparing Your Mind and Body

Seeing auras requires a relaxed, focused state of mind. Before you begin any practice session, take a few moments to center yourself. Find a comfortable seated position and close your eyes. Take several deep breaths, inhaling slowly through your nose and exhaling through your mouth. As you breathe, imagine tension leaving your body with each exhale.

Once you feel relaxed, bring your attention to the space between your eyebrows, often referred to as the third eye. This area is associated with intuition and psychic abilities in many spiritual traditions. Gently focus on this spot for a few moments, imagining it opening like a flower, enhancing your ability to perceive subtle energies.

The Soft Gaze Technique

One of the most effective techniques for beginners is the soft gaze method. This approach involves looking at your subject without focusing too hard, allowing your peripheral vision to come into play. Here's how to practice:

1. Choose your subject - a willing friend, a plant, or even your own hand against a plain background.

2. Look at the subject, but instead of focusing directly on them, gaze slightly to the side or just above their head.

3. Relax your eyes and let your vision soften. It might feel a bit like you're daydreaming or looking through the subject rather than at them.

4. Pay attention to the space around the subject. Don't try to force yourself to see anything; simply observe with a relaxed, open mind.

5. You might start to notice a faint outline or a subtle change in the air around the subject. This could appear as a hazy glow, a slight color change, or a shimmer in the air.

6. If your eyes start to strain or water, take a break. Look away, blink a few times, and then try again.

Remember, patience is key here. When I first started, it took me several sessions before I saw anything at all. And even then, it was just a faint, colorless haze. But with consistent practice, that haze gradually became clearer and more colorful.

The Peripheral Vision Method

Another effective technique utilizes your peripheral vision, which is more sensitive to subtle changes in light and movement. Here's how to practice:

1. Position your subject about 3-4 feet in front of you against a plain background.

2. Focus on a point just above the subject's head or slightly to the side.

3. Without moving your eyes, pay attention to what you can see in your peripheral vision. You might notice a faint glow or color around the edges of the subject.

4. If you see something, resist the urge to look directly at it. The moment you shift your focus, the aura might seem to disappear. This is because your peripheral vision is picking up on subtle energy that your direct vision might miss.

5. Practice holding this peripheral gaze for a few minutes at a time, taking breaks as needed.

This method can be particularly effective because our peripheral vision is connected to different parts of our brain than our central vision. It's often able to pick up on subtle energies that we might not consciously register when looking directly at something.

The Blink Technique

The blink technique is a simple yet powerful method that can help you catch glimpses of the aura. Here's how it works:

1. Set up your subject against a plain background in a dimly lit room.

2. Look at the subject and blink rapidly for about 30 seconds to a minute.

3. After the rapid blinking, hold your eyes open and gaze softly at the subject.

4. You might notice an afterimage or a subtle glow around the subject. This is often the first layer of the aura becoming visible to you.

5. If you don't see anything at first, try blinking rapidly again and then holding your gaze steady.

The theory behind this technique is that the rapid blinking helps to reset and refresh your visual perception, making it easier to notice subtle changes in the energy field around the subject.

Practicing with Your Hands

One of the easiest ways to start seeing auras is to practice with your own hands. This method is great because you always have your practice subject with you! Here's how to do it:

1. Find a comfortable seated position in a dimly lit room with a plain background.

2. Hold your hands out in front of you, palms facing each other about 6 inches apart.

3. Slowly move your hands closer together and then further apart, maintaining a soft gaze on the space between your palms.

4. As you do this, you might start to notice a faint mist or strings of energy between your hands. This is the beginning of perceiving your own energy field.

5. Once you can consistently see this energy between your palms, try expanding your awareness to the area around your entire hand.

I remember the first time I tried this technique. I was skeptical at first, but after a few minutes of practice, I began to see what looked like a faint, smoke-like substance between my palms. It was a thrilling moment that encouraged me to keep practicing and developing my skills.

Using Nature as Your Teacher

Nature can be an excellent teacher when it comes to seeing auras. Plants, in particular, are great subjects for beginners because they have a vibrant energy field and they stay perfectly still for you. Here's how to practice with plants:

1. Choose a healthy plant with broad leaves. Place it against a plain, light-colored background in a room with soft, natural light.

2. Sit comfortably about 3-4 feet away from the plant.

3. Using the soft gaze technique, look at the edges of the leaves.

4. You might start to notice a faint, greenish-white glow around the edges of the leaves. This is the plant's aura becoming visible to you.

5. Once you can consistently see this glow, try expanding your perception to the entire plant.

Working with plants can be a wonderfully grounding experience. Not only are you developing your aura-seeing abilities, but you're also connecting with the natural world in a profound way.

Overcoming Common Challenges

As you embark on this journey of learning to see auras, you're likely to encounter some challenges. Let's address some of the most common ones and how to overcome them:

1. Impatience: It's natural to want to see results quickly, but rushing the process can actually hinder your progress. Remember that learning to see auras is a skill that takes time to develop. Be patient with yourself and enjoy the journey.

2. Self-doubt: You might find yourself questioning whether you're really seeing an aura or just imagining it. This self-doubt can block your progress. Trust your perceptions, even if they seem faint or unclear at first. With practice, your confidence will grow.

3. Eye strain: Trying too hard to see auras can lead to eye strain and headaches. Always practice in short sessions (10-15 minutes) and take breaks if you feel any discomfort.

4. Inconsistent results: Some days you might see auras clearly, while other days you might struggle to see anything at all. This is normal and doesn't mean you're losing your ability. Many factors, including your energy levels, mood, and environment, can affect your perception.

5. Difficulty distinguishing colors: In the beginning, you might only see a colorless glow. This is a great start! As you continue to practice, you'll gradually begin to perceive colors. Don't try to force it; let the colors come naturally as your perception develops.

Integrating Aura Viewing into Daily Life

As you develop your ability to see auras, you can start integrating this skill into your daily life. Here are some ways to practice throughout your day:

1. Observe people in public spaces: While waiting in line at the grocery store or sitting on public transport, practice using your peripheral vision to observe the energy fields of those around you. Remember to be respectful and discreet.

2. Connect with nature: When you're out for a walk, try perceiving the auras of trees, flowers, or even animals if they'll sit still long enough for you.

3. Check in with your own aura: Use a mirror to practice seeing your own aura. This can be a powerful tool for self-awareness and personal growth.

4. Practice with friends and family: As you become more confident in your abilities, ask willing friends or family members to be subjects for your practice.

Remember, the key to developing this skill is consistent practice. Even just a few minutes each day can lead to significant improvements over time.

Keeping an Aura Journal

One practice that I've found incredibly helpful in my own journey is keeping an aura journal. After each practice session, take a few moments to write down what you experienced. Note any colors, shapes, or sensations you perceived, as well as any challenges you faced or breakthroughs you had.

This journal serves several purposes:

1. It helps you track your progress over time, which can be encouraging when you're facing challenges.

2. It allows you to notice patterns in your experiences, which can provide valuable insights into your developing abilities.

3. It serves as a record of your journey that you can look back on with pride as your skills improve.

4. Writing about your experiences helps to reinforce them in your mind, potentially enhancing your ability to perceive auras in the future.

Understanding What You're Seeing

As you begin to consistently see auras, you might wonder what the different colors and patterns mean. While we'll dive deeper into aura interpretation in the next chapter, it's helpful to have a basic understanding of what you're seeing.

The colors you perceive in an aura can provide insights into a person's emotional state, energy levels, and even aspects of their personality. For example, a bright, clear aura generally indicates good health and positive energy, while a dull or muddy aura might suggest fatigue or emotional distress.

You might also notice that auras aren't always uniform. They can have different colors in different areas, layers of color, or even patterns like spots or stripes. All of these variations can provide additional information about the person's energy field.

Remember, though, that aura reading is a complex skill that goes beyond just seeing colors. As you continue to develop your abilities, you'll learn to interpret the subtleties of what you're perceiving.

The Role of Intuition

As you practice seeing auras, you'll likely find that your intuition plays a significant role in the process. Sometimes, you might "sense" or "feel" an aura before you actually see it with your eyes. This is a normal part of the process and is worth paying attention to.

Your intuition can provide valuable insights that complement what you're seeing visually. For example, you might visually perceive a person's aura as predominantly blue, but intuitively sense a underlying current of anxiety. Both pieces of information are valuable in understanding the person's energy field.

Don't be afraid to trust your intuitive impressions as you practice. They're an important part of developing your overall ability to perceive and interpret auras.

The Importance of Grounding

As you develop your ability to see auras, it's crucial to maintain a strong connection to the physical world. This practice, known as grounding, helps to balance your energy and prevent you from becoming overwhelmed by the subtle energies you're learning to perceive.

After each practice session, take a few moments to ground yourself. You can do this by:

1. Visualizing roots growing from your feet deep into the earth.

2. Eating a small snack, preferably something healthy and substantial like nuts or fruit.

3. Taking a short walk outside, paying attention to the sensation of your feet on the ground.

4. Holding a grounding crystal like black tourmaline or hematite.

Grounding helps to integrate your experiences and ensures that you're not neglecting your physical well-being as you develop your psychic abilities.

Embracing the Journey

As we conclude this chapter, I want to encourage you to embrace the journey of learning to see auras. Remember that every person's path is unique. Some might see auras clearly after just a few practice sessions, while others might take weeks or even months to start perceiving energy fields consistently.

Whatever your experience, know that the very act of practicing is expanding your awareness and opening you up to the subtle energies that surround us all. Even if you're not seeing auras as clearly as you'd like yet, you're developing a heightened sensitivity to energy that can enrich your life in numerous ways.

Continue to practice regularly, stay patient with yourself, and maintain an attitude of curiosity and openness. Before long, you'll find that the invisible world of energy becomes as real and tangible to you as the physical world you navigate every day.

In our next chapter, we'll explore how to move beyond just seeing auras to sensing and feeling them with your other senses. This multi-sensory approach will deepen your understanding of energy fields and enhance your overall ability to work with auras. But for now, take some time to practice the techniques we've covered in this chapter. Remember, the key to success is consistent, patient practice. Trust the process, and most importantly, enjoy the journey of discovery that lies ahead.

Chapter 6 - Beyond Seeing: Sensing and Feeling Auras

As we journey deeper into the world of aura perception, we find ourselves moving beyond the realm of visual cues and into a more subtle, yet equally powerful, domain of sensory experience. In this chapter, we'll explore the myriad ways you can perceive auras through senses other than sight, focusing primarily on feeling and sensing energy fields. These techniques not only complement visual aura reading but can also stand alone as valuable tools for understanding and interacting with the energetic world around us.

The Multi-Sensory Nature of Aura Perception

When I first began my journey into aura work, I was fixated on the idea of seeing colorful energy fields around people. It wasn't until I met my mentor, Sarah, that I realized how limiting this perspective was. "Energy speaks to us in many languages," she told me. "Some hear it as music, others feel it as texture or temperature. Your job is to discover which language resonates with you."

This insight opened up a whole new world of possibilities for me, and I hope it does the same for you. As we explore these alternative methods of aura perception, remember that each person's experience is unique. You may find that you're naturally inclined towards one method over others, or that a combination of techniques works best for you.

Feeling Auras: The Art of Energetic Touch

One of the most direct ways to perceive an aura is through the sense of touch – not physical touch, but energetic touch. This method involves using your hands to feel the energy field surrounding a person or object.

To begin, find a willing partner or a plant (plants are excellent subjects for practicing energy work). Stand about arm's length away and close your eyes. This removes visual distractions and allows you to focus on your other senses. Slowly extend your hands towards your subject, palms facing them. As you do this, pay close attention to any sensations you feel in your palms and fingers.

You might experience:

- Warmth or coolness

- Tingling or buzzing

- Pressure or resistance

- A feeling of thickness or density in the air

These sensations indicate that you're interacting with the subject's energy field. With practice, you'll learn to distinguish between different qualities of energy and what they might mean.

I remember the first time I successfully felt an aura. I was practicing with a friend who had just finished an intense workout. As my hands approached her body, I felt a distinct warmth and a slight pulsing sensation, almost like feeling a heartbeat from a distance. It was subtle but unmistakable, and it left me in awe of the energetic exchanges happening around us all the time.

Mapping the Aura Through Sensation

Once you've become comfortable sensing the general presence of an aura, you can begin to map out its structure and characteristics. Start at the outer edges of the energy field and slowly move your hands closer to the subject's body. Pay attention to how the sensations change as you move through different layers of the aura.

You might notice:

- Areas where the energy feels denser or more active
- Spots that seem cooler or warmer than others
- Regions where you experience resistance or a pulling sensation

These variations can provide insights into the subject's energetic state. For example, a area of intense warmth might indicate increased energy flow or activity, while a cool spot could suggest blocked or stagnant energy.

Interpreting Energetic Sensations

As you develop your ability to feel auras, you'll start to create your own "dictionary" of sensations and their meanings. However, here are some common interpretations to get you started:

Warmth: Often associated with areas of high energy flow, healing, or emotional openness.

Coolness: May indicate areas of low energy, blocked chakras, or emotional guardedness.

Tingling: Can suggest active energy movement, often related to healing or spiritual awakening.

Pressure or resistance: Might point to energetic blockages or areas of tension.

Pulsing: Could indicate strong emotional or physical energy centers.

Remember, these are general guidelines. Your personal experiences and intuitions are equally valid and important in interpreting what you feel.

Developing Your Energetic Touch

Like any skill, feeling auras improves with practice. Here are some exercises to help you develop your energetic touch:

1. Self-practice: Start by feeling your own aura. Run your hands over different parts of your body, staying a few inches away from your skin. Notice how the sensations differ between areas.

2. Nature connection: Practice with plants or trees. They have strong, stable energy fields that are often easier to sense than human auras when you're starting out.

3. Partner work: Take turns with a friend, practicing feeling each other's auras. Discuss your experiences and see if your perceptions match how the other person is feeling.

4. Blind tests: Have someone hold an object behind a screen, and try to describe its energy without seeing it. This helps build confidence in your abilities.

5. Energetic scanning: Practice "scanning" a room or space with your hands, noting any areas where the energy feels different.

Beyond Touch: Other Ways of Sensing Auras

While feeling auras with your hands is a powerful technique, it's not the only way to sense energy fields without relying on sight. Let's explore some other methods that might resonate with you.

Empathic Sensing

Some people have a natural ability to sense the emotional states of others. This empathic ability can be a form of aura reading. When you enter a room, pay attention to any sudden shifts in your own emotional state. These could be reflections of the auras around you.

For instance, you might suddenly feel anxious in a room full of stressed people, or uplifted when you're near someone with a particularly positive energy. With practice, you can learn to distinguish between your own emotions and those you're picking up from others.

Intuitive Knowing

Sometimes, information about a person's aura or energy state comes to you as a sudden insight or "knowing." This might manifest as a clear thought, a mental image, or a gut feeling about the person's state of being.

I once had a client who came in for a healing session. Before she even spoke, I had a strong sense that she was dealing with grief. This insight turned out to be accurate – she had recently lost a close family member. My intuitive knowing had picked up on the energetic signature of her emotional state.

Auditory Perception

Some individuals report hearing auras as tones, music, or even words. This might sound like a high-pitched ringing for vibrant energy, a low hum for grounded energy, or even specific musical notes associated with different parts of the aura.

If you're musically inclined, you might find this method particularly accessible. Try sitting quietly and "listening" to the energy around you. What do you hear?

Gustatory and Olfactory Sensing

Although less common, some people experience tastes or smells associated with different auras. You might taste sweetness when encountering a loving energy, or smell something unpleasant when faced with negative energy.

These experiences are often fleeting and subtle, so it requires practice and attention to notice and interpret them. Keep an open mind and pay attention to any unusual tastes or smells that occur when you're focusing on someone's energy.

Synesthesia and Aura Perception

It's worth noting that some people experience a neurological phenomenon called synesthesia, where stimulation of one sensory or cognitive pathway leads to involuntary experiences in another pathway. For instance, someone might always see a specific color when they hear a certain musical note.

If you have synesthesia, you might find that it plays a role in how you perceive auras. Your unique sensory associations could provide an additional layer of information when sensing energy fields.

Trusting Your Perceptions

As you explore these various methods of sensing auras, you might find yourself doubting your experiences. "Am I really feeling something, or is it just my imagination?" This is a common concern, and it's important to address it.

The truth is, the line between imagination and subtle energy perception can be blurry, especially when you're starting out. However, consistently practicing and recording your experiences will help you distinguish between the two.

I encourage you to keep a journal of your aura sensing experiences. Note down what you perceive, any insights you receive, and how these correlate with what you know about the person or situation. Over time, you'll likely see patterns emerge that validate your perceptions.

Remember, even experienced aura readers sometimes question their abilities. The key is to approach your practice with an attitude of curious exploration rather than skeptical doubt. Trust that your abilities will develop and refine over time.

Integrating Multiple Sensing Techniques

As you become more comfortable with various methods of aura perception, you'll likely find that you naturally integrate multiple techniques. You might start by visually scanning an aura, then use your hands to feel for areas of interest, and finally tune in empathically to get a sense of the emotional energy.

This multi-sensory approach can provide a rich, nuanced understanding of a person's energy field. It's like assembling a puzzle – each sensing technique contributes a piece, and together they form a comprehensive picture.

Ethical Considerations in Aura Sensing

As we delve deeper into these powerful techniques, it's crucial to discuss the ethical implications of aura sensing. Remember, when you're perceiving someone's aura, you're essentially accessing personal information about them. This ability comes with responsibility.

Always ask for permission before reading someone's aura, and respect their privacy. Some people might not be comfortable with having their energy field examined, and that's okay. Additionally, be mindful of how you share the information you perceive. Approach it with sensitivity and compassion, understanding that you're dealing with deeply personal aspects of someone's being.

Practical Applications of Non-Visual Aura Sensing

Now that we've explored various techniques for sensing auras beyond sight, let's consider how you might apply these skills in practical ways:

1. Personal well-being: Regularly check in with your own aura using these techniques. This can help you identify and address energetic imbalances before they manifest as physical or emotional issues.

2. Healing work: If you're a healer or therapist, these sensing techniques can provide valuable insights into your clients' energetic states, helping you tailor your treatments more effectively.

3. Interpersonal relationships: Understanding the energy dynamics between yourself and others can help you navigate relationships more smoothly. You'll be better equipped to recognize when someone needs support or when it might be best to give them space.

4. Environmental awareness: Use your sensing abilities to assess the energy of spaces. This can be particularly helpful when choosing a new home, setting up a workspace, or creating a healing environment.

5. Decision making: Tuning into the energy of a situation can provide additional information to guide your choices. Trust your gut feelings – they're often your energy-sensing abilities at work.

Overcoming Challenges in Aura Sensing

As with any skill, you may encounter challenges as you develop your ability to sense auras. Here are some common obstacles and strategies to overcome them:

Inconsistent results: Don't be discouraged if your perceptions seem to vary from day to day. Our sensitivity to energy can be affected by many factors, including our own emotional state, physical health, and environmental conditions. Regular practice will help stabilize your abilities.

Difficulty interpreting sensations: Keep a record of your experiences and look for patterns over time. This will help you develop your personal "energy vocabulary."

Energetic overwhelm: If you find yourself feeling drained or overwhelmed after practicing aura sensing, it's important to learn grounding and shielding techniques (which we'll cover in later chapters). Remember, it's okay to take breaks and pace yourself.

Self-doubt: It's natural to question your abilities, especially when dealing with subtle energies. Validate your experiences by sharing them with like-minded individuals or joining a development circle for energy workers.

The Journey of Sensory Expansion

As we conclude this chapter, I want to emphasize that developing your ability to sense auras is a journey of expanding your sensory awareness. It's about learning to tune into the subtle energies that are always around us but often go unnoticed in our busy daily lives.

This journey requires patience, practice, and an open mind. Some days, you might feel like you're making great progress, while on others, it might seem like you can't sense anything at all. This is all part of the process. Trust in your innate ability to perceive energy and keep exploring.

Remember, every person's experience with sensing auras is unique. The techniques and interpretations I've shared in this chapter are meant to be guidelines, not rigid rules. As you practice, you'll develop your own methods and understanding of what different sensations mean to you.

In our next chapter, we'll explore how disruptions in the aura can occur and what causes them. This knowledge will be crucial as we move towards learning how to heal and maintain a healthy energy field. But for now, I encourage you to spend some time practicing the techniques we've discussed. Explore how you uniquely sense and interpret the energy around you. You might be surprised at the depth of information available when you tune in to the world beyond visual perception.

Remember, the ability to sense auras is not just a skill – it's a way of experiencing the world more fully, of tapping into the interconnected web of energy that links us all. As you develop this ability, you may find that it opens up new dimensions of understanding and connection in your life. Embrace this journey with curiosity and wonder, and trust in your growing ability to navigate the unseen world of energy that surrounds us all.

Chapter 7 - Common Aura Disruptions and Their Causes

As we delve deeper into the realm of aura healing, it's crucial to understand that our energy fields are not impervious to damage or disturbance. Just as our physical bodies can experience illness or injury, our auras can become disrupted, depleted, or imbalanced. In this chapter, we'll explore the various ways in which our energy fields can be affected and the underlying causes of these disruptions.

The Delicate Nature of Our Energy Fields

Before we dive into the specific disruptions that can occur in our auras, it's important to recognize the inherently sensitive nature of our energy fields. Your aura is constantly interacting with the world around you, absorbing and exchanging energy with your environment and the people you encounter. This dynamic interaction is what allows you to experience life fully, but it also leaves your aura vulnerable to various influences.

Think of your aura as a beautiful, iridescent bubble surrounding you. While it's resilient in many ways, it can also be easily affected by external forces. Just as a soap bubble can be distorted by a gust of wind or burst when it comes into contact with a sharp object, your aura can be similarly impacted by the energies and experiences you encounter in your daily life.

Environmental Factors Affecting Your Aura

One of the most common sources of aura disruption comes from our immediate environment. The spaces we inhabit and the energies present in those spaces can have a profound effect on our energy fields.

Electromagnetic Fields (EMFs): In our modern world, we're constantly surrounded by electronic devices that emit electromagnetic radiation. While the debate about the long-term health effects of EMFs continues, many energy workers and sensitives report that prolonged exposure to these fields can create disturbances in the aura. You might have noticed feeling drained after spending hours in front of a computer or experiencing headaches when using your smartphone for extended periods. These symptoms could be indicative of EMF-related aura disruption.

Negative Energy in Physical Spaces: Have you ever walked into a room and immediately felt uncomfortable or uneasy? This sensation is often attributed to the presence of negative energy that has accumulated in that space. Such energy can come from past arguments, prolonged stress, or even traumatic events that occurred there. When you spend time in these environments, your aura can absorb some of this negative energy, leading to disruptions in your own energy field.

Natural Disasters and Earth Changes: Major environmental events like earthquakes, storms, or even significant changes in weather patterns can have an impact on our auras. These events often release intense energies that can be overwhelming for our energy fields. You might find yourself feeling unusually anxious or unsettled during these times, which could be a sign that your aura is responding to these powerful natural forces.

Emotional Trauma and Its Impact on Your Energy Field

Our emotional experiences play a significant role in shaping our auras. Traumatic events, in particular, can leave lasting imprints on our energy fields.

Sudden Emotional Shocks: Unexpected negative events like the loss of a loved one, a sudden breakup, or receiving bad news can create immediate disruptions in your aura. These shocks can cause your energy field to contract rapidly, sometimes leaving it in a state of contraction long after the initial event has passed.

Prolonged Stress and Anxiety: While acute emotional events can cause sudden disruptions, chronic stress and anxiety can lead to gradual but persistent changes in your aura. Over time, these emotional states can cause your aura to become dim, frayed, or develop weak spots. You might notice that during particularly stressful periods in your life, you feel more vulnerable to external energies or find it harder to maintain your emotional balance.

Unresolved Past Traumas: Even if you've consciously moved on from past traumatic experiences, unresolved emotions related to these events can continue to affect your aura. These unhealed wounds can manifest as dark spots or tears in your energy field, often corresponding to the chakras most closely associated with the type of trauma experienced.

Physical Illness and Its Relationship to Aura Health

The state of our physical health is intimately connected to the condition of our auras. In fact, many energy healers believe that disruptions in the aura often precede physical manifestations of illness.

Chronic Illnesses: Long-term health conditions can create persistent disturbances in your energy field. These disruptions might appear as areas of discoloration, cloudiness, or even gaps in your aura. Conversely, maintaining a healthy aura through energy healing practices can sometimes help alleviate symptoms of chronic conditions by supporting your body's natural healing processes.

Acute Illnesses and Injuries: When you experience a sudden illness or injury, you might notice rapid changes in your aura. These can include temporary holes or weak spots in your energy field, often concentrated around the affected area of your physical body. As you recover physically, you'll likely find that your aura also begins to heal and strengthen.

Substance Abuse and Poor Lifestyle Choices: The choices we make regarding our physical health can have profound effects on our auras. Substance abuse, poor diet, lack of exercise, and insufficient sleep can all lead to a weakened and depleted energy field. You might experience this as a general sense of being drained or more susceptible to negative energies.

Psychic Attacks and Energy Vampirism

While it's important not to become paranoid, it's also crucial to acknowledge that sometimes, disruptions in our auras can come from the intentional or unintentional actions of others.

Intentional Negative Energy: In rare cases, individuals might deliberately direct negative energy towards you. This is often referred to as a psychic attack. While the effectiveness of such attacks is debatable, many sensitive individuals report feeling drained, anxious, or experiencing unusual bad luck when targeted in this way. These experiences are often attributed to disruptions in the aura caused by the directed negative energy.

Energy Vampirism: More common than intentional psychic attacks is the phenomenon of energy vampirism. This occurs when individuals, often unconsciously, drain energy from those around them. You might have encountered people who leave you feeling exhausted after interacting with them. This drain on your energy can create temporary or even lasting disruptions in your aura if you're frequently exposed to such individuals.

Toxic Relationships: Relationships characterized by constant conflict, manipulation, or emotional abuse can have severe impacts on your aura. These toxic connections can create persistent weak spots in your energy field, making you more vulnerable to further disruptions and negative energies.

Spiritual and Energetic Practices Gone Wrong

Ironically, sometimes our attempts to work with energy can lead to disruptions in our auras if not done correctly or with proper protection.

Improper Grounding: When engaging in spiritual or energetic practices, it's crucial to properly ground yourself. Failure to do so can leave your aura overstimulated or unbalanced. You might experience this as feeling "spacey," disconnected from reality, or emotionally volatile after spiritual work.

Overexposure to High-Frequency Energies: While working with high-frequency energies can be beneficial, overexposure without proper preparation can overwhelm your energy field. This can lead to temporary disruptions in your aura, manifesting as feelings of disorientation or even physical symptoms like headaches or nausea.

Incomplete Energy Clearings: When attempting to clear negative energy from your aura, it's important to complete the process fully. Incomplete clearings can sometimes leave residual negative energy trapped in your field, potentially causing more harm than if you hadn't attempted the clearing at all.

Recognizing Aura Disruptions

Now that we've explored the various causes of aura disruptions, you might be wondering how to recognize when your own energy field has been affected. While some individuals can visually perceive auras and their disturbances, most of us need to rely on other cues.

Physical Symptoms: Disruptions in your aura often manifest as physical sensations. You might experience unexplained fatigue, headaches, dizziness, or a general feeling of being unwell. Some people report feeling a heaviness in certain parts of their body or unusual aches and pains that don't seem to have a physical cause.

Emotional Indicators: Pay attention to your emotional state. Sudden mood swings, persistent feelings of anxiety or depression, or difficulty controlling your emotions can all be signs of aura disruption. You might also find yourself feeling unusually vulnerable to the emotions of others, as if you're absorbing their feelings more than usual.

Energetic Sensations: If you're attuned to subtle energies, you might directly feel disturbances in your aura. This could manifest as a sense of pressure or tingling in certain areas around your body, or a feeling of your personal space being invaded even when no one is physically close to you.

Intuitive Knowing: Sometimes, you might simply have a strong intuition that something is off with your energy field. Trust these instincts, as they often stem from your subconscious awareness of changes in your aura.

Behavioral Changes: Disruptions in your aura can sometimes lead to changes in your behavior. You might find yourself acting out of character, making decisions that don't align with your values, or struggling with habits and patterns you thought you had overcome.

The Importance of Regular Aura Maintenance

Given the many ways our auras can become disrupted, it's clear that regular maintenance of our energy fields is crucial for our overall well-being. Just as we engage in daily hygiene practices for our physical bodies, we should also develop habits that support the health of our auras.

Daily Grounding Practices: Start your day with a simple grounding exercise. This could be as easy as visualizing roots growing from your feet into the earth, drawing up stabilizing energy. This practice helps to anchor your aura and make it more resilient to potential disruptions throughout the day.

Regular Energy Cleansing: Incorporate energy cleansing techniques into your routine. This might involve smudging with sage, taking salt baths, or using visualization techniques to clear your aura of any accumulated negative energy. By doing this regularly, you prevent minor disruptions from building up into more significant issues.

Mindful Interactions: Be conscious of the energy you're exchanging in your daily interactions. Before entering potentially stressful situations or meeting with individuals who tend to drain your energy, take a moment to reinforce your aura's boundaries. You can do this through visualization, affirming your energetic sovereignty, or using protective symbols or crystals.

Balanced Lifestyle Choices: Remember that everything you do affects your aura. Strive to maintain a balanced lifestyle with proper nutrition, regular exercise, sufficient sleep, and stress-management practices. These foundational habits support the overall health and resilience of your energy field.

Regular Check-ins: Set aside time periodically to check in with your aura. This could be through meditation, working with a trusted energy healer, or using tools like aura photography. Regular assessments can help you catch and address minor disruptions before they become more significant issues.

Conclusion: Empowerment Through Awareness

As we conclude this exploration of common aura disruptions and their causes, I want to emphasize that knowledge is power. By understanding the various ways your energy field can be affected, you're taking the first step towards more effective protection and healing of your aura.

Remember, experiencing disruptions in your aura is not a sign of failure or weakness. It's a natural part of navigating life as an energetic being in a complex world. What matters is how you respond to these disruptions and the steps you take to maintain and restore the health of your energy field.

In the following chapters, we'll delve deeper into specific techniques for cleansing, repairing, and strengthening your aura. You'll learn practical tools to address the disruptions we've discussed here and to cultivate a vibrant, resilient energy field that supports your overall well-being.

As we move forward, carry with you the awareness you've gained in this chapter. Let it inform your interactions with the world around you and your approach to your own energetic health. Your aura is a precious part of your being, deserving of care, attention, and respect. By honoring and tending to your energy field, you're nurturing the very essence of who you are.

Chapter 8 - The Physical Manifestation of Aura Problems

As we delve deeper into the intricate world of aura healing, it's crucial to understand how disruptions in our energy field can manifest as physical symptoms and illnesses. In this chapter, we'll explore the profound connection between the health of our aura and our bodily well-being. I'll guide you through the various ways in which aura problems can affect your physical health, and how addressing these energetic imbalances can lead to improved overall wellness.

The Mind-Body-Energy Connection

Before we dive into the specific physical manifestations of aura problems, it's important to establish the fundamental relationship between our energy field, our mind, and our physical body. These three aspects of our being are inextricably linked, constantly influencing and affecting one another.

Think of your aura as a protective bubble that surrounds your physical body. This energetic shield not only contains your own energy but also acts as a filter for external energies. When your aura is healthy and balanced, it helps maintain your physical and emotional well-being. However, when disruptions occur in your energy field, they can eventually trickle down to affect your physical body.

I often explain this concept to my clients using the analogy of a computer system. Your physical body is like the hardware, your mind is the software, and your aura is the firewall and operating system that manages everything. When a virus penetrates the firewall, it can corrupt the software and eventually damage the hardware. Similarly, when your aura is compromised, it can lead to mental and emotional disturbances, which in turn can manifest as physical symptoms.

Common Physical Symptoms of Aura Disruptions

Now that we've established the connection between your aura and physical health, let's explore some of the most common ways that energetic imbalances can manifest in your body. As you read through these, you might recognize some symptoms you've experienced but never attributed to your energy field before.

Fatigue and Low Energy

One of the most prevalent physical manifestations of aura problems is persistent fatigue and low energy levels. When your energy field is depleted or damaged, it can struggle to properly distribute life force energy throughout your body. This can leave you feeling drained, even after a full night's sleep.

I once worked with a client, Sarah, who complained of constant exhaustion despite maintaining a healthy lifestyle. Upon examining her aura, I discovered significant tears in her energy field, particularly around her solar plexus chakra. These tears were causing a continuous leak of her vital energy. Once we began repairing her aura, Sarah noticed a dramatic improvement in her energy levels within just a few weeks.

Headaches and Migraines

Frequent headaches or migraines can often be linked to disruptions in the upper layers of your aura, particularly those associated with your crown and third eye chakras. These disruptions can create energetic congestion or blockages, which can manifest as pain in your head.

I remember a case where a man named Michael had been suffering from chronic migraines for years. Traditional medical treatments had provided little relief. When we examined his aura, we found a dense, dark energy accumulated around his crown chakra. Through targeted aura cleansing and repair techniques, we were able to dissipate this energy, leading to a significant reduction in the frequency and intensity of his migraines.

Digestive Issues

The state of your aura can have a surprising impact on your digestive system. Imbalances or blockages in the lower chakras, particularly the solar plexus chakra, can manifest as various digestive issues such as bloating, constipation, or irritable bowel syndrome (IBS).

I've worked with numerous clients who've experienced relief from chronic digestive problems after addressing issues in their aura. One client, Emma, had been struggling with IBS for years. When we examined her energy field, we found that her solar plexus chakra was severely constricted, affecting the flow of energy to her digestive organs. Through chakra balancing and aura repair techniques, Emma was able to find significant relief from her symptoms.

Skin Problems

Your skin, as the largest organ of your body, often reflects the state of your aura. Persistent skin issues like acne, eczema, or unexplained rashes can sometimes be traced back to disruptions in your energy field, particularly in the outer layers of your aura.

I once worked with a teenager, Alex, who had been battling severe acne for years. Traditional treatments had shown limited success. When we looked at his aura, we found that the outer layers were clouded with stagnant energy, particularly around his face and neck. By focusing on cleansing and repairing these outer layers, Alex saw a noticeable improvement in his skin condition.

Weakened Immune System

A compromised aura can lead to a weakened immune system, making you more susceptible to frequent colds, flu, and other infections. Your aura acts as an energetic immune system, and when it's not functioning optimally, your physical immune system can suffer as a result.

I recall a client, Lisa, who seemed to catch every bug that was going around. Her aura examination revealed numerous weak spots and tears, allowing negative energies to easily penetrate her energy field. After dedicated work on strengthening and repairing her aura, Lisa found that she fell ill much less frequently.

Chronic Pain

Persistent pain in specific areas of the body can often be linked to energetic blockages or disturbances in the corresponding parts of your aura. For example, chronic back pain might be associated with issues in the aura around your back chakras.

One of my clients, Robert, had been suffering from chronic shoulder pain for years. Medical examinations had found no physical cause for his discomfort. When we looked at his aura, we discovered a dense knot of energy around his shoulder area. Through focused energy work to dissolve this knot and repair the surrounding aura, Robert experienced significant relief from his long-standing pain.

The Subtle Onset of Physical Symptoms

It's important to understand that the physical manifestation of aura problems often occurs gradually. Your energy field acts as a buffer, absorbing and processing various energies before they reach your physical body. This means that disruptions in your aura may not immediately result in physical symptoms.

Think of it like a pool with a slow leak. At first, you might not notice any change in the water level. But over time, if the leak isn't addressed, the water level will noticeably drop. Similarly, small disruptions in your aura might not cause immediate physical issues, but if left unaddressed, they can accumulate and eventually manifest as physical symptoms or illness.

This gradual onset is one reason why many people don't immediately connect their physical symptoms to the state of their energy field. It's also why regular aura maintenance and cleansing are so important – they can help prevent these small disruptions from building up over time.

The Role of Emotions in Physical Manifestations

When discussing the physical manifestations of aura problems, we can't overlook the crucial role that emotions play in this process. Our emotional state has a profound impact on our aura, and consequently, on our physical health.

Negative emotions like anger, fear, or sadness can create disturbances in our energy field. If these emotions are intense or persistent, they can lead to more significant disruptions in our aura. These energetic disturbances can then manifest as physical symptoms.

For instance, prolonged stress or anxiety can create a constriction in your aura, particularly around your heart and solar plexus chakras. This constriction can manifest physically as tension in your chest, shortness of breath, or even heart palpitations.

I worked with a client, Jennifer, who was experiencing frequent panic attacks. When we examined her aura, we found that it was extremely constricted around her heart and throat chakras, reflecting her unexpressed fears and anxieties. As we worked on releasing these emotional blockages and expanding her aura, Jennifer found that her panic attacks became less frequent and less intense.

The Aura as an Early Warning System

One of the most fascinating aspects of the aura-body connection is that disruptions in your energy field often precede physical symptoms. This means that your aura can serve as an early warning system for potential health issues.

By learning to tune into your aura and recognize subtle changes in your energy field, you can potentially identify and address health issues before they manifest physically. This is one of the many reasons why developing your ability to sense and interpret your own aura can be so valuable for your overall health and well-being.

I often encourage my clients to practice regular aura self-checks. By taking a few moments each day to tune into your energy field, you can become more aware of any changes or disturbances. These might manifest as feelings of heaviness in certain areas, color changes in your aura (if you're able to see auras), or simply a sense that something is "off" energetically.

The Healing Journey: From Energy to Physical

Understanding the connection between your aura and your physical health is just the first step. The real power lies in using this knowledge to facilitate healing. When you address disruptions in your energy field, you're not just healing your aura – you're also creating the conditions for physical healing to occur.

This healing journey often follows a pattern:

1. Identify the energetic disruption
2. Clear and repair the affected areas of the aura
3. Balance and strengthen the overall energy field
4. Observe the gradual alleviation of physical symptoms

It's important to note that while aura healing can be incredibly powerful, it should not replace conventional medical treatment.

Instead, it can work in harmony with traditional healthcare, supporting and enhancing your body's natural healing processes.

I always advise my clients to maintain open communication with their healthcare providers while undertaking energy work. In many cases, a holistic approach that combines conventional medicine with energy healing can yield the best results.

Case Study: A Holistic Healing Journey

To illustrate how this process works in practice, let me share the story of one of my clients, David. When David first came to me, he was suffering from chronic fatigue syndrome (CFS). He had been dealing with debilitating exhaustion for over two years, and despite numerous medical tests and treatments, had found little relief.

When we examined David's aura, we found several issues:

1. His overall energy field was extremely depleted, appearing dim and contracted.

2. There were significant tears in the lower layers of his aura, particularly around his root and sacral chakras.

3. His solar plexus chakra was almost completely closed, blocking the flow of energy to the rest of his body.

4. There was a dense, grey energy accumulated around his heart chakra, reflecting unprocessed grief and emotional pain.

We developed a comprehensive aura healing plan for David, which included:

1. Regular energy cleansing sessions to remove the stagnant and negative energy from his field.

2. Targeted repair work to mend the tears in his aura, particularly focusing on the root and sacral chakras to help him feel more grounded and secure.

3. Chakra balancing exercises, with special attention to opening and energizing his solar plexus chakra.

4. Emotional release techniques to help process the grief stored in his heart chakra.

5. Teaching David daily practices to maintain and strengthen his aura, including visualization exercises and energy protection techniques.

David committed to this healing plan, combining it with the treatments recommended by his doctor. Over the course of several months, we saw significant improvements:

1. David's energy levels gradually increased, allowing him to engage in more daily activities without exhaustion.

2. The tears in his aura began to heal, and his overall energy field became brighter and more expansive.

3. His solar plexus chakra opened up, improving his energy flow and digestion.

4. As we worked through the emotional energy around his heart chakra, David reported feeling more emotionally balanced and resilient.

5. Most importantly, David's physical symptoms of CFS began to alleviate. While he still had some low-energy days, they became less frequent, and he was able to return to many of the activities he had given up due to his condition.

David's story illustrates how addressing issues in the aura can lead to improvements in physical health, especially when combined with appropriate medical care. It's a powerful reminder of the intricate connection between our energy field and our physical well-being.

Preventive Aura Care for Physical Health

While much of this chapter has focused on how aura problems can manifest as physical symptoms, it's equally important to consider the preventive aspect of aura care. By maintaining a healthy, balanced energy field, you can potentially ward off physical ailments before they take hold.

Think of caring for your aura as a form of energetic hygiene, much like brushing your teeth or washing your hands. Regular aura maintenance can help keep your energy field strong and resilient, better able to withstand the various energetic challenges we face in daily life.

Some simple practices for preventive aura care include:

1. Daily aura cleansing: This can be as simple as visualizing a shower of white light washing away any negative or stagnant energy from your field.

2. Grounding exercises: Regularly connecting with the earth's energy can help stabilize and strengthen your aura, particularly the lower chakras.

3. Energy protection techniques: Learning to create a protective shield around your aura can help prevent energy drain and deflect negative influences.

4. Chakra balancing: Regular attention to the health of your chakras can help maintain a smooth flow of energy throughout your aura.

5. Mindful living: Being aware of the energetic impact of your thoughts, emotions, and surroundings can help you make choices that support the health of your aura.

By incorporating these practices into your daily routine, you're not just caring for your energy field — you're also taking proactive steps to support your physical health.

The Journey of Holistic Healing

As we conclude this chapter, I want to emphasize that the relationship between your aura and your physical health is a two-way street. Just as disruptions in your energy field can manifest as physical symptoms, improvements in your aura can lead to enhanced physical well-being.

Understanding this connection opens up a whole new dimension of healing possibilities. It invites us to approach health and wellness from a truly holistic perspective, one that acknowledges the intricate dance between energy and matter, between the seen and the unseen aspects of our being.

As you continue your journey into aura healing, I encourage you to pay close attention to how changes in your energy field correlate with changes in your physical health. You may be surprised at the connections you discover, and the potential for healing that unfolds.

Remember, every step you take to heal and strengthen your aura is a step towards greater physical vitality and overall well-being. In the next chapter, we'll explore specific techniques for emotional healing through aura work, further deepening your understanding of the profound connections between your energy field and your total health.

Chapter 9 - Emotional Healing and Your Aura

Our emotional experiences play a crucial role in shaping our energy field, and in turn, our aura significantly influences our emotional well-being. In this chapter, we'll explore the intricate relationship between emotions and the aura, and delve into powerful techniques for addressing emotional wounds that affect your energy field. We'll also discuss practices for releasing trapped emotions and healing past traumas, all with the goal of restoring balance and vitality to your aura.

The Emotional-Aura Connection

As you've learned in previous chapters, your aura is a reflection of your overall state of being, including your physical, mental, and emotional health. When it comes to emotions, your aura acts as both a mirror and a sponge. It reflects your current emotional state, but it also absorbs and stores emotional energy from past experiences.

Think of a time when you were feeling particularly joyful or excited. If you could see your aura at that moment, you'd likely notice it expanding and radiating bright, vibrant colors. Conversely, during times of sadness or anger, your aura might appear contracted, dull, or murky. This is the immediate reflection of your emotional state in your energy field.

But what about those emotions that linger long after the initial experience? That's where the sponge-like quality of your aura comes into play. Intense emotional experiences, especially traumatic ones, can leave lasting imprints on your energy field. These imprints can manifest as distortions, dark spots, or even tears in your aura.

I once worked with a client, let's call her Sarah, who had been through a difficult divorce. Years after the event, she still struggled with feelings of worthlessness and fear of abandonment. When we examined her aura, we found a persistent dark, muddy patch in her heart chakra area. This was the energetic manifestation of her unresolved emotional pain.

Identifying Emotional Wounds in Your Aura

Before we can begin the healing process, it's essential to identify where emotional wounds are affecting your aura. While you may not be able to visually see your aura (though if you've been practicing the techniques from Chapter 5, you might!), there are other ways to sense these disturbances:

1. Physical sensations: Pay attention to areas of your body where you frequently feel tension, pain, or discomfort. These can often correlate with emotional blockages in your aura.

2. Emotional patterns: Notice recurring emotional reactions that seem disproportionate to current situations. These may be clues to past wounds still affecting your energy field.

3. Intuitive awareness: As you become more attuned to your energy, you might develop an intuitive sense of where your aura feels "off" or imbalanced.

4. Professional aura reading: Consider seeking out a trained aura reader who can provide insights into the state of your energy field.

Techniques for Releasing Trapped Emotions

Once you've identified areas of emotional stagnation in your aura, it's time to begin the process of release. Here are some powerful techniques to help you let go of trapped emotions:

1. Emotional Freedom Technique (EFT):
   EFT, also known as tapping, is a powerful tool for releasing emotional blockages. It involves tapping on specific acupressure points while focusing on the emotional issue at hand. This technique helps to clear the energy pathways in your body and aura, allowing trapped emotions to be released.

To practice EFT, start by identifying the emotion you want to address. Rate its intensity on a scale of 0-10. Then, while focusing on this emotion, use your fingertips to tap about 7 times on each of the following points:

- The top of your head

- The inner edge of your eyebrow

- The outer corner of your eye

- Under your eye

- Under your nose

- Your chin

- Your collarbone

- Under your arm (about 4 inches below your armpit)

As you tap, repeat a phrase that acknowledges the emotion and affirms your self-acceptance, such as "Even though I feel this anger, I deeply and completely accept myself." After a full round of tapping, reassess the intensity of the emotion. Repeat the process until you feel a significant reduction in the emotional charge.

2. Breathwork:
    Your breath is a powerful tool for moving energy through your body and aura. Deep, intentional breathing can help dislodge stuck emotions and clear your energy field. Try this simple technique:

Sit comfortably and close your eyes. Take a few normal breaths to center yourself. Then, imagine the emotion you want to release as a color or texture in your aura. As you inhale deeply through your nose, visualize clean, pure energy entering your body and aura. As you exhale forcefully through your mouth, see the colored emotion being expelled from your energy field. Continue this for 5-10 minutes, or until you feel a sense of release.

3. Journaling:

    Writing can be a cathartic way to process and release emotions. Set aside time to write freely about your feelings, without judgment or censorship. As you write, imagine the emotions flowing out of you and onto the page. When you're done, you can choose to keep the writing or, if it feels right, destroy it as a symbolic act of release.

4. Sound healing:

    Sound vibrations can help break up stagnant emotional energy in your aura. You can use your own voice, singing bowls, or even recorded sound frequencies. One simple technique is to use vowel sounds:

Stand with your feet hip-width apart and take a few deep breaths. Then, starting with your root chakra, work your way up through your energy centers, making the following sounds:

- Root chakra: "Uh" (as in "cup")

- Sacral chakra: "Ooo" (as in "you")

- Solar plexus chakra: "Oh" (as in "go")

- Heart chakra: "Ah" (as in "father")

- Throat chakra: "Eye" (as in "fly")

- Third eye chakra: "Aye" (as in "say")

- Crown chakra: "Eee" (as in "see")

As you make each sound, visualize the vibration clearing any emotional blockages from that area of your aura.

Healing Past Traumas

While the techniques above can be effective for everyday emotional release, healing deeper traumas often requires a more focused approach. Here are some methods for addressing and healing past traumas that may be affecting your aura:

1. Inner Child Work:
   Many of our deepest emotional wounds stem from childhood experiences. Inner child work involves connecting with and nurturing the part of you that still carries those early hurts. Here's a simple visualization to get started:

Close your eyes and take a few deep breaths. Imagine yourself in a safe, peaceful place. Now, visualize your younger self – the child who experienced the trauma or pain – appearing before you. Notice how they look, what they're wearing, and how they're feeling. Approach this younger version of yourself with compassion and love. Ask them what they need from you. Listen carefully to their response. Then, provide whatever comfort or reassurance they need. This might involve hugging them, speaking words of love and acceptance, or simply being present with them. As you do this, visualize healing light surrounding both you and your inner child, repairing any damage to your shared aura.

2. Timeline Therapy:
   This technique involves revisiting past events to release their emotional charge and reframe your perspective. Here's how to do it:

Sit comfortably and close your eyes. Imagine a timeline stretching out before you, representing your life from birth to the present moment. Locate the traumatic event on this timeline. Float above the timeline and move to a point just before the trauma occurred. As you watch the event unfold, notice it as if you're watching a movie. Observe without judgment, allowing any emotions to arise and pass. Now, imagine floating to a point after the event. Look back and ask yourself what lessons or strengths you gained from this experience. Finally, return to the present moment, bringing with you any new insights or perspectives. As you do this, visualize your aura becoming clearer and brighter, free from the weight of the past trauma.

3. Forgiveness Work:
   Holding onto resentment or anger can create significant distortions in your aura. Forgiveness – of others and yourself – is a powerful way to heal these distortions. Remember, forgiveness doesn't mean condoning harmful actions; it's about freeing yourself from the burden of negative emotions.

To practice forgiveness, start by identifying who you need to forgive (including yourself, if applicable). Write a letter to this person, expressing all your feelings about what happened. Then, write a response from their perspective, imagining what they might say. Finally, write a letter of forgiveness, releasing both them and yourself from the emotional burden. As you do this, visualize the dark or distorted areas of your aura associated with this situation beginning to clear and heal.

4. Energy Psychology Techniques:
   Methods like EMDR (Eye Movement Desensitization and Reprocessing) and AIT (Advanced Integrative Therapy) can be powerful tools for processing traumatic memories and healing their impact on your energy field. These techniques often involve bilateral stimulation (alternating left-right movements or taps) while focusing on the traumatic memory. This helps to reprocess the memory and reduce its emotional charge.

While it's best to work with a trained professional for these methods, you can try a simple bilateral stimulation technique at home:

Sit comfortably and think of the traumatic event. Notice where you feel it in your body and what emotions arise. Rate the intensity of your distress on a scale of 0-10. Then, while holding the memory in mind, tap alternately on your right and left knees (or shoulders) for about a minute. Take a deep breath and reassess your distress level. Repeat the process until you feel a significant reduction in emotional intensity.

Integrating Emotional Healing into Daily Life

Healing emotional wounds and their impact on your aura is not a one-time event, but an ongoing process. Here are some ways to incorporate emotional healing into your daily life:

1. Regular energy cleansing:
   Make it a habit to cleanse your aura daily, especially after emotionally charged experiences. You can use techniques like smudging with sage, taking a salt bath, or simply visualizing a waterfall of light washing over your energy field.

2. Emotional check-ins:
   Set aside time each day to check in with your emotions. How are you feeling? Where do you feel it in your body? Are there any areas of your aura that feel heavy or blocked? This awareness can help you address emotional issues before they become deeply entrenched in your energy field.

3. Mindfulness practice:
   Developing a regular mindfulness or meditation practice can help you become more aware of your emotions as they arise, allowing you to process them in real-time rather than suppressing them.

4. Physical movement:
   Activities like yoga, dance, or even just stretching can help move emotional energy through your body and aura. Pay attention to any emotions that arise during physical movement and allow them to flow through you.

5. Gratitude practice:
   Focusing on gratitude can help shift your emotional state and brighten your aura. Each day, take time to acknowledge three things you're grateful for, no matter

how small.

6. Creative expression:
   Engaging in creative activities like art, music, or writing can be a powerful way to process emotions and heal your aura. Allow yourself to create freely, without judgment, as a form of emotional release.

When to Seek Professional Help

While the techniques in this chapter can be powerful tools for emotional healing and aura repair, there may be times when professional help is necessary. Consider seeking support from a therapist, energy healer, or other qualified professional if:

- You're dealing with severe trauma or deep-seated emotional issues

- You feel overwhelmed by your emotions or unable to cope

- You're experiencing persistent depression, anxiety, or other mental health concerns

- You're not seeing progress despite consistent self-healing efforts

- You feel stuck or unsure how to proceed in your healing journey

Remember, seeking help is a sign of strength, not weakness. A skilled professional can provide valuable insights and techniques to support your emotional healing and aura repair process.

Conclusion: The Ongoing Journey of Emotional Healing

As we conclude this chapter, I want you to remember that emotional healing is a journey, not a destination. Just as our physical bodies require ongoing care and maintenance, so too do our emotional selves and our auras. The techniques we've explored here are tools you can return to again and again as you navigate life's emotional landscape.

Each time you release a trapped emotion or heal a past wound, you're not just improving your current emotional state – you're also clearing and strengthening your aura, creating a more resilient energy field that can better support you in the future. This work ripples out, affecting not just your own well-being, but also your interactions with others and your impact on the world around you.

As we move forward into the next chapter on cleansing techniques for removing negative energy, remember that emotional healing and energy cleansing go hand in hand. The clearer your aura becomes through emotional healing, the more effective other cleansing techniques will be. And as you remove negative energy from your aura, you'll find it easier to access and heal deeper emotional layers.

Your emotional health and the state of your aura are intimately connected, each influencing and reflecting the other. By tending to both with care and intention, you're creating a foundation for holistic well-being that encompasses all aspects of your being – physical, emotional, mental, and spiritual. Trust in this process, be patient with yourself, and know that with each step, you're moving towards a more vibrant, balanced, and authentic expression of your true self.

Chapter 10 - Cleansing Techniques: Removing Negative Energy

As we journey through life, our auras inevitably accumulate negative energy. This buildup can occur from various sources: stressful experiences, toxic relationships, challenging environments, or even our own negative thoughts and emotions. Just as we cleanse our physical bodies, it's crucial to regularly purify our energy fields. In this chapter, we'll explore a variety of effective techniques for cleansing your aura of negative or stagnant energy.

Understanding the Need for Aura Cleansing

Before we dive into specific cleansing methods, it's important to understand why regular aura cleansing is necessary. Think of your aura as a sponge, constantly absorbing energy from your surroundings. Over time, this sponge can become saturated with heavy, negative energies that weigh you down emotionally, mentally, and even physically.

You might notice signs that your aura needs cleansing: feeling constantly drained, experiencing unexplained mood swings, or sensing a general heaviness in your being. These are indicators that it's time to give your energy field some attention and care.

I remember a time when I felt unusually irritable and lethargic for weeks. No matter how much I slept or how well I ate, I couldn't shake the feeling of being weighed down. It wasn't until I performed a thorough aura cleansing that I felt a sudden lightness and clarity. The difference was so stark that it reinforced for me the importance of regular energetic maintenance.

Setting the Stage for Cleansing

Before you begin any cleansing technique, it's crucial to create the right environment and mindset. Find a quiet, comfortable space where you won't be disturbed. Take a few deep breaths to center yourself and set a clear intention for your cleansing session. You might say something like, "I intend to release all negative and stagnant energy from my aura, making space for positivity and light."

Remember, the power of intention is significant in energy work. Your focused will amplifies the effectiveness of any technique you use. Approach your cleansing practice with an open heart and a belief in its potential to create positive change.

Smudging: An Ancient Purification Practice

One of the most well-known and widely practiced aura cleansing techniques is smudging. This ancient practice involves burning sacred herbs or resins and using the smoke to purify your energy field. The most commonly used herb for smudging is white sage, known for its potent cleansing properties.

To smudge yourself, light a bundle of dried sage until it produces a steady stream of smoke. As the smoke rises, use your hand or a feather to guide it around your body, starting at your feet and moving upward. As you do this, visualize the smoke carrying away any negative energy clinging to your aura.

I often use smudging when I feel the need for a quick energy reset. The earthy scent of sage immediately grounds me, and I can almost feel the negativity dissolving as the smoke envelops me. It's a simple yet powerful practice that I encourage you to try.

Other herbs and resins can be used for smudging as well, each with its unique properties:

- Palo Santo: Known as "holy wood," it's excellent for inviting positive energy after cleansing.

- Lavender: Calming and soothing, ideal for emotional healing.

- Cedar: Grounding and protective, often used for space clearing.

- Frankincense: Purifying and elevating, it can help raise your spiritual vibration.

Experiment with different smudging materials to find what resonates best with you. Remember, it's not just about the physical act of burning these herbs; it's about the intention and reverence you bring to the practice.

Sound Healing: Vibrational Cleansing

Sound is a powerful tool for aura cleansing, capable of breaking up stagnant energy and restoring harmony to your energy field. The vibrations produced by certain instruments can penetrate your aura, dislodging negative energy and realigning your own energetic frequency.

One of the most effective sound healing tools is the Tibetan singing bowl. The rich, resonant tones produced by these bowls create sound waves that wash over your aura, cleansing it much like water cleanses your physical body. To use a singing bowl for aura cleansing, simply strike or rim the bowl and allow the sound to envelop you. As you listen, visualize the sound waves moving through your energy field, dissolving any areas of negativity or stagnation.

Other sound healing tools include:

- Tuning forks: These can be used to target specific areas of your aura that feel blocked or heavy.

- Drums: The rhythmic beating of a drum can help shake loose negative energy and realign your own energetic rhythms.

- Chimes or bells: The clear, high-pitched tones can cut through dense energy and bring a sense of lightness to your aura.

You don't need to be a skilled musician to benefit from sound healing. Even humming or chanting simple tones can have a cleansing effect on your aura. I often use the vowel sounds (A, E, I, O, U) as a quick cleansing technique when I'm feeling energetically off-balance.

Visualization Exercises: The Power of Your Mind

Never underestimate the power of your own mind in cleansing your aura. Visualization exercises can be incredibly effective in removing negative energy and restoring balance to your energy field. These exercises harness the power of your imagination and intention to create real energetic shifts.

One simple yet powerful visualization is the "White Light Shower." Here's how to do it:

1. Close your eyes and take a few deep breaths to center yourself.

2. Imagine a bright, pure white light above your head.

3. Visualize this light pouring down over you like a shower, starting at the crown of your head and flowing all the way down to your feet.

4. As the light flows over you, see it washing away any dark, heavy, or negative energy from your aura.

5. Imagine this negative energy being absorbed by the earth, where it's neutralized and transformed.

6. Continue this visualization until you feel clean, light, and refreshed.

I often use this technique before bed or upon waking, as it helps me start and end my day with a clean energetic slate. The beauty of visualization exercises is that you can do them anywhere, at any time, without any special tools or preparation.

Another effective visualization is the "Aura Combing" technique:

1. Visualize your aura as a luminous egg-shaped field surrounding your body.

2. Imagine you have a large, golden comb in your hand.

3. Starting at the top of your aura, visualize combing downward, seeing the comb catch and remove any dark or sticky energy.

4. Continue combing all around your aura, front, back, and sides.

5. See the removed energy dissolving into the earth.

This technique can be particularly helpful if you're feeling energetically "tangled" or confused. The act of combing can bring a sense of order and clarity to your energy field.

Salt Baths: Soaking Away Negativity

Water has long been recognized for its cleansing and purifying properties, not just for the physical body but for the energy body as well. A salt bath is a wonderful way to cleanse your aura, especially when you're feeling overwhelmed or emotionally drained.

Epsom salt, sea salt, or Himalayan pink salt can all be used for this purpose. These salts are believed to draw out negative energy and replace it with beneficial minerals. To prepare a cleansing salt bath:

1. Fill your bathtub with warm water.

2. Add 1-2 cups of your chosen salt to the water.

3. If desired, add a few drops of essential oils like lavender (for relaxation) or eucalyptus (for purification).

4. As you soak in the bath, visualize the salt water drawing out all negative energy from your aura.

5. See this energy being neutralized by the salt and washed away down the drain.

I find salt baths particularly effective after I've been in crowded places or had challenging interactions with others. The combination of warm water, salt, and focused intention leaves me feeling energetically lighter and more centered.

If you don't have access to a bathtub, you can achieve a similar effect with a foot soak. Simply fill a basin with warm water and salt, and soak your feet for 15-20 minutes while visualizing the cleansing process.

Crystals for Aura Cleansing

Crystals are powerful tools for energy work, and certain stones are particularly effective for aura cleansing. These crystals can absorb negative energy from your aura and help to realign your energy field. Some of the most potent crystals for aura cleansing include:

- Clear Quartz: Known as the "master healer," it can cleanse and amplify energy.

- Black Tourmaline: Excellent for grounding and protection, it absorbs negative energy.

- Selenite: A high-vibration stone that cleanses and charges the aura.

- Amethyst: Purifies the aura and transmutes negative energy into positive.

To use crystals for aura cleansing, you can simply hold them in your hands during meditation, place them on your body while lying down, or pass them through your aura (similar to the smudging technique). As you work with the crystal, visualize it drawing out any negative or stagnant energy from your aura.

I keep a piece of black tourmaline on my desk to continuously cleanse my energy field throughout the day. When I need a more intensive cleansing, I'll lie down with a clear quartz at my crown chakra and a piece of black tourmaline at my feet, allowing their energies to flow through my aura for about 15-20 minutes.

Remember to cleanse your crystals regularly, as they accumulate the negative energy they absorb. You can do this by leaving them in moonlight, burying them in the earth, or using sound or smudging to clear them.

Nature's Cleansing Power

Never underestimate the cleansing power of nature. Spending time outdoors can be one of the most effective ways to purify your aura. The natural world is filled with clean, high-vibration energy that can help to reset and recharge your own energy field.

Here are some ways to harness nature's cleansing power:

Earthing: Walking barefoot on grass, sand, or soil allows you to directly connect with the Earth's energy. This practice, also known as "grounding," can help to neutralize negative energy in your aura and replace it with the Earth's stable, nurturing energy.

Tree Hugging: It may sound cliché, but embracing a tree can be a powerful aura cleansing technique. Trees are natural energy conduits, drawing energy from the earth and sky. When you hug a tree, you align your energy with this natural flow, which can help to clear and balance your aura.

Ocean or River Cleansing: Water in its natural state has a strong cleansing effect on the aura. Standing in the ocean or a flowing river, visualize the water washing away any negative energy from your aura. The negative ions produced by moving water also contribute to this cleansing effect.

Sunlight and Moonlight Bathing: Both the sun and moon offer unique energies that can cleanse and recharge your aura. Spend time in direct sunlight (being mindful of skin protection) or moonlight, visualizing the light penetrating and purifying your energy field.

I make it a point to spend time in nature regularly, even if it's just a short walk in a local park. The shift in my energy is always noticeable – I feel clearer, more grounded, and more in tune with myself after these nature "baths."

Breath Work for Aura Cleansing

Your breath is a powerful tool that's always available to you for aura cleansing. Specific breathing techniques can help to release stagnant energy and invite fresh, vital energy into your aura. Here's a simple yet effective breathing exercise for aura cleansing:

1. Find a comfortable seated position and close your eyes.

2. Take a few normal breaths to center yourself.

3. Inhale deeply through your nose, visualizing clean, bright energy entering your aura.

4. Hold the breath for a moment, seeing this energy permeate your entire energy field.

5. Exhale forcefully through your mouth, imagining all negative energy being expelled from your aura.

6. Repeat this process for 5-10 minutes, or until you feel a noticeable shift in your energy.

This technique, often called "cleansing breath," can be particularly helpful in moments of stress or when you feel suddenly impacted by negative energy. I often use it before important meetings or after challenging conversations to quickly reset my energy field.

Another powerful breathing technique is alternate nostril breathing, or Nadi Shodhana in yoga practice. This technique balances the left and right hemispheres of the brain and can help to harmonize your energy field:

1. Use your right thumb to close your right nostril.

2. Inhale deeply through your left nostril.

3. Close your left nostril with your ring finger, release your thumb, and exhale through your right nostril.

4. Inhale through the right nostril.

5. Close the right nostril, release your ring finger, and exhale through the left nostril.

6. This completes one cycle. Repeat for 5-10 minutes.

Regular practice of these breathing techniques can help maintain a clean and balanced aura, making you more resilient to negative energies in your environment.

The Power of Intention and Affirmations

While we've explored many external tools and techniques for aura cleansing, it's crucial to remember the power of your own thoughts and intentions. Your aura responds to your mental and emotional state, so cultivating positive thoughts and intentions can be a form of continuous aura cleansing.

Affirmations are positive statements that can help to shift your energy and cleanse your aura. Here are some affirmations you might use:

"I release all negative energy from my aura."
"My energy field is clear, bright, and vibrant."
"I am surrounded by positive, healing energy."
"I easily deflect and transmute negative energy."

Repeat these affirmations daily, especially when you feel your energy becoming heavy or clouded. The key is to say them with conviction and to truly feel the truth of these statements as you speak them.

You can also set intentions for your aura's cleanliness and protection. Each morning, take a moment to set an intention like, "Today, I intend to maintain a clear and protected aura." This simple act can make you more mindful of your energy throughout the day and more proactive in maintaining its cleanliness.

Creating a Cleansing Ritual

Now that we've explored various aura cleansing techniques, I encourage you to create your own cleansing ritual. This could be a daily practice or something you do weekly or whenever you feel the need for energetic cleansing.

Your ritual might look something like this:

1. Begin with a few minutes of centering breath work.

2. Light a sage smudge stick and cleanse your aura with the smoke.

3. Use a singing bowl or play some cleansing music.

4. Sit quietly and visualize white light showering over your aura.

5. Hold a cleansing crystal like clear quartz or black tourmaline.

6. End with some positive affirmations for aura health.

The specifics of your ritual will depend on what resonates most with you. The important thing is to approach it with intention and consistency. Over time, you'll likely notice that maintaining a clean aura becomes easier, and you'll be more sensitive to when your energy field needs attention.

Maintaining a Clean Aura

Aura cleansing isn't just about removing negative energy – it's also about maintaining that clean state. Here are some tips for keeping your aura clear and vibrant:

Practice Mindfulness: Be aware of your thoughts and emotions throughout the day. Negative thoughts can cloud your aura, so catch them early and transform them into positive ones.

Energy Protection: Before entering crowded or potentially negative environments, visualize a protective shield around your aura. This can help prevent the absorption of unwanted energies.

Regular Energy Checks: Take a moment each day to tune into your aura. How does it feel? Is it light and expansive, or heavy and contracted? This awareness will help you address issues before they become significant.

Healthy Lifestyle: Your physical health impacts your aura. Maintain a balanced diet, exercise regularly, and ensure you're getting enough rest.

Limit Exposure to Negativity: While we can't always control our environment, we can limit our exposure to sources of negative energy, whether that's certain people, places, or media.

Practice Gratitude: Cultivating an attitude of gratitude raises your vibration and naturally cleanses your aura. Try keeping a gratitude journal or simply noting things you're thankful for throughout the day.

By incorporating these practices into your daily life, you create an environment where your aura can thrive, making it more resilient to negative influences.

Conclusion: Your Journey to a Cleaner, Brighter Aura

As we conclude this chapter, I want to emphasize that aura cleansing is a personal journey. What works best for you may be different from what works for others. The techniques we've explored – from smudging and sound healing to visualization and crystal work – are all valuable tools, but the most powerful tool is your own intention and commitment to maintaining your energetic health.

Remember, your aura is constantly interacting with the world around you. It's natural for it to accumulate some negative energy over time. Regular cleansing isn't about achieving perfection; it's about maintaining balance and vitality in your energy field.

As you continue to practice these techniques, you'll likely become more attuned to your own energy. You'll start to notice subtle shifts in your aura and be able to address imbalances more quickly. This heightened awareness is a beautiful side effect of regular aura maintenance.

In our next chapter, we'll build on these cleansing techniques to explore more advanced methods of aura repair, focusing on addressing tears and holes in the energy field. But for now, I encourage you to experiment with the cleansing methods we've discussed. Pay attention to how you feel before and after each practice. With time and consistency, you'll discover which techniques resonate most deeply with you, allowing you to create a personalized aura cleansing practice that keeps your energy field clear, bright, and resilient.

Remember, caring for your aura is an act of self-love. By maintaining a clean and vibrant energy field, you're not only benefiting yourself but also positively influencing the world around you. Your cleansed and balanced aura becomes a beacon of light, contributing to the collective energy in a beautiful and meaningful way.

Chapter 11 - Repairing Tears and Holes in Your Energy Field

As we delve into the intricate world of aura healing, we arrive at a crucial juncture – the repair of tears and holes in your energy field. These disruptions in your aura can have profound effects on your overall well-being, and learning to address them is an essential skill for anyone on the path of energetic self-care.

Understanding Aura Damage

Before we dive into the repair techniques, it's important to understand what we're dealing with. Imagine your aura as a beautiful, luminous egg-shaped field surrounding your body. Now, picture what happens when this delicate structure sustains damage. Tears can appear as jagged rips or frayed edges in your energy field, while holes might manifest as dark spots or voids where your aura's natural radiance is diminished.

These imperfections in your aura aren't just cosmetic – they can leave you feeling drained, vulnerable to negative energies, and disconnected from your spiritual essence. You might experience this as a persistent feeling of being "off," or notice that you're more susceptible to others' moods and energies than usual.

I remember when I first became aware of a significant tear in my own aura. It was after a period of intense stress and emotional turmoil. I felt constantly fatigued, and it seemed like every little setback hit me harder than it should. It wasn't until I worked with an experienced energy healer that I realized the extent of the damage to my energy field – and more importantly, that it could be repaired.

Identifying Aura Damage

Before you can repair your aura, you need to locate the areas that need attention. This process requires a blend of intuition and practiced perception. Here are some ways you can identify tears and holes in your energy field:

1. Visual Perception: If you've developed the ability to see auras, look for areas where the color appears faded, dark, or discontinuous. Tears might look like actual rips in the fabric of your energy, while holes could appear as dark spots or voids.

2. Kinesthetic Sensing: Even if you can't see auras, you can often feel them. Run your hands a few inches above your body, paying attention to any areas that feel different. Cold spots, tingling sensations, or a feeling of emptiness could indicate damage.

3. Emotional Mapping: Our emotions are closely tied to our energy field. Pay attention to any emotions that feel stuck or overwhelming. These might correspond to areas of aura damage.

4. Physical Symptoms: Sometimes, aura damage manifests as physical discomfort. Unexplained aches, persistent fatigue in specific body parts, or a feeling of heaviness could all be signs of energetic disruption.

5. Intuitive Knowing: Trust your intuition. You might have a sudden insight or a persistent feeling about a particular area of your aura needing attention. Don't dismiss these hunches — they're often your higher self guiding you towards healing.

Preparing for Aura Repair

Once you've identified the areas of damage, it's time to prepare for the healing process. Creating the right environment and mindset is crucial for effective aura repair. Here's how you can set the stage for healing:

1. Create a Sacred Space: Choose a quiet, comfortable area where you won't be disturbed. This could be a dedicated meditation space or simply a cleared corner of a room. The key is to feel safe and relaxed in this environment.

2. Cleanse the Area: Use sage, palo santo, or incense to cleanse the energy of your chosen space. As you do this, set the intention for healing and protection.

3. Ground Yourself: Before working with your aura, it's essential to be firmly grounded. You can do this by visualizing roots growing from your feet deep into the earth, or by spending a few moments in nature before your healing session.

4. Raise Your Vibration: Engage in activities that elevate your energy before attempting repairs. This could include listening to uplifting music, practicing gratitude, or doing

some gentle yoga or stretching.

5. Set Your Intention: Clearly state your intention for healing. You might say something like, "I intend to repair and strengthen my aura, restoring it to its natural state of wholeness and vitality."

Techniques for Repairing Tears

Now that we're prepared, let's explore some powerful techniques for repairing tears in your aura. Remember, healing is a personal process, so feel free to adapt these methods to suit your unique needs and intuition.

1. Visualization Healing

One of the most effective ways to repair aura tears is through focused visualization. Here's a step-by-step process you can follow:

a) Close your eyes and take several deep, calming breaths.

b) Visualize your aura as a luminous egg-shaped field surrounding your body.

c) Locate the tear in your mind's eye. See it clearly, noting its size, shape, and any associated colors or sensations.

d) Imagine a warm, healing light emanating from your heart center. This light is the color that feels most healing to you – it might be golden, pink, blue, or pure white.

e) Direct this healing light towards the tear. See it gently knitting the edges of the tear back together, like a cosmic needle and thread.

f) As the tear closes, visualize the area becoming stronger, more vibrant, and more resilient than before.

g) Once the repair is complete, see your entire aura glowing with renewed strength and vitality.

h) Take a few more deep breaths, feeling gratitude for this healing, before gently opening your eyes.

2. Energy Weaving

This technique involves using your hands to literally 'weave' energy back into place:

a) Sit comfortably and center yourself with a few deep breaths.

b) Raise your hands to the area of your aura where you've identified a tear.

c) Using your dominant hand, make small, circular motions as if you're gathering energy.

d) With your other hand, make weaving motions, as if you're patching the tear with this gathered energy.

e) Continue this process, feeling the energy becoming denser and more cohesive as you work.

f) When you feel the tear has been repaired, smooth your hands over the area, sealing the work you've done.

3. Sound Healing

Sound vibrations can be incredibly powerful for aura repair. You can use your own voice or tools like singing bowls or tuning forks:

a) Choose a sound that resonates with you – this could be a specific tone, a mantra, or a healing song.

b) Direct this sound towards the torn area of your aura.

c) Visualize the sound waves interacting with your energy field, their vibrations gently closing the tear.

d) Continue until you feel a shift in the energy of the affected area.

Healing Holes in Your Aura

Holes in your aura require a slightly different approach than tears. These voids need to be filled with fresh, vibrant energy. Here are some techniques to address aura holes:

1. Energy Infusion

This technique involves channeling healing energy to fill the void:

a) Locate the hole in your aura through visualization or sensing.

b) Imagine a fountain of pure, healing light above your head.

c) See this light pouring down through your crown chakra, filling your entire being.

d) Direct this light specifically to the area with the hole.

e) Visualize the light filling the void, restoring the natural radiance of your aura.

f) Continue until you feel the area is fully saturated with this healing energy.

2. Crystal Healing

Crystals can be powerful allies in repairing aura holes:

a) Choose a crystal that resonates with you for healing. Clear quartz is an excellent all-purpose choice, but trust your intuition if drawn to a specific stone.

b) Cleanse and charge the crystal with your intention for healing.

c) Lie down comfortably and place the crystal on or near the area of your aura that needs repair.

d) Visualize the crystal's energy expanding, filling the hole in your aura with its pure, healing vibration.

e) Leave the crystal in place for at least 15 minutes, or until you intuitively feel the process is complete.

3. Color Therapy

Color can be a potent tool for aura repair:

a) Determine which color you feel is needed to heal the hole. This might be the color you associate with that area of your aura, or a color that intuitively feels right.

b) Visualize this color as a concentrated beam of light.

c) Direct this colored light into the hole in your aura.

d) See the color expanding to fill the entire void, restoring vibrancy to your energy field.

e) Once the hole is filled, visualize the color integrating seamlessly with the rest of your aura.

Advanced Techniques for Persistent Damage

Sometimes, aura damage can be stubborn, resisting our initial attempts at repair. In these cases, we need to dig a little deeper and employ more advanced techniques. These methods often involve addressing the root causes of the damage and may require more time and patience.

1. Timeline Healing

This technique involves journeying back to the moment when the damage occurred:

a) Enter a deep meditative state.

b) Visualize a timeline of your life, stretching out before and behind you.

c) Ask your higher self to guide you to the point on this timeline when the aura damage occurred.

d) Once there, observe the event without judgment. What happened? How did it affect your energy?

e) From your current perspective, send healing energy to your past self at this moment.

f) Visualize this healing energy repairing the damage in real-time, altering the trajectory of your energy field from that point forward.

g) See this healing rippling forward through time, restoring your aura in the present moment.

2. Soul Retrieval

Sometimes, aura damage is associated with soul loss – parts of our essence that have become disconnected due to trauma. This advanced technique aims to reintegrate these lost aspects:

a) In a meditative state, set the intention to connect with any lost soul fragments.

b) Visualize yourself in a safe, sacred space – this could be a beautiful garden, a serene beach, or any place that feels secure and nurturing to you.

c) Call out to your lost soul parts, inviting them to return if they're ready.

d) If any parts appear, approach them with love and compassion. Listen to what they need to feel safe returning.

e) When a soul part is ready, welcome it back, visualizing it reintegrating with your energy field and filling any voids in your aura.

f) Express gratitude for this reunion and the healing it brings.

3. Karmic Cord Cutting

Sometimes, aura damage is linked to unhealthy energetic connections with others. This technique helps sever these ties:

a) In meditation, scan your aura for any cords connecting you to other people, places, or past events.

b) For each cord, assess whether it's serving your highest good. If not, it's time to release it.

c) Visualize yourself lovingly and firmly cutting this cord with an energetic blade of light.

d) As the cord is severed, see both ends being sealed with healing light.

e) Feel the relief and lightness as these connections are released, and visualize your aura becoming brighter and more cohesive.

Maintaining Your Repaired Aura

Once you've done the work of repairing tears and holes in your aura, it's crucial to maintain this restored state. Here are some practices to keep your energy field strong and resilient:

1. Daily Energy Hygiene: Just as you shower to keep your physical body clean, engage in daily practices to cleanse your energy field. This could include visualization exercises, smudging with sage, or taking salt baths.

2. Regular Grounding: Stay connected to the earth's healing energy by spending time in nature, walking barefoot on grass or sand, or visualizing roots growing from your feet into the earth.

3. Mindful Living: Be aware of the environments and people you expose yourself to. Choose to spend time in uplifting places and with individuals who respect your energy boundaries.

4. Energetic Protection: Before entering potentially draining situations, visualize a protective bubble or shield around your aura.

5. Chakra Balancing: Regularly check in with and balance your chakras, as they play a crucial role in the overall health of your aura.

6. Self-Care: Nurture yourself on all levels – physical, emotional, mental, and spiritual. A well-cared-for self naturally maintains a stronger aura.

7. Continuous Learning: Stay curious about energy work. The more you understand about your own energy field, the better equipped you'll be to maintain its health.

When to Seek Professional Help

While these techniques can be incredibly powerful for self-healing, there may be times when professional help is beneficial. Consider seeking the assistance of an experienced energy healer if:

1. You're dealing with severe or long-standing aura damage that resists self-healing efforts.

2. You're working through significant trauma or deep-seated emotional issues that are affecting your energy field.

3. You feel overwhelmed by the energy healing process or unsure of how to proceed.

4. You're experiencing persistent physical symptoms alongside aura issues.

5. You simply feel guided to work with a professional for additional support and insight.

Remember, seeking help is a sign of strength, not weakness. Sometimes, an outside perspective can provide the breakthrough we need in our healing journey.

As we conclude this chapter on repairing tears and holes in your energy field, I want to remind you of the incredible resilience of your aura. Just like your physical body, your energy field has an innate capacity for healing. The techniques we've explored here are tools to support and enhance this natural process.

Trust in your ability to heal, be patient with yourself, and approach this work with an open heart and mind. Every step you take towards repairing and strengthening your aura is a step towards greater wholeness, vitality, and spiritual connection.

In our next chapter, we'll explore how crystals can be powerful allies in your ongoing aura care, providing specific guidance on selecting and using these earth treasures for energetic healing. But for now, take some time to practice the techniques we've covered here. Your aura – and your entire being – will thank you for this loving attention.

Chapter 12 - Crystal Healing for Aura Repair

As we journey deeper into the realm of aura healing, we come across one of the most enchanting and powerful tools at our disposal: crystals. These beautiful, natural wonders have been revered for centuries for their healing properties, and their ability to interact with our energy fields is truly remarkable. In this chapter, we'll explore how to harness the power of crystals to repair, strengthen, and balance your aura.

The Magic of Crystals: More Than Just Pretty Rocks

When I first stumbled upon crystal healing, I was skeptical. How could these seemingly ordinary stones have any effect on my energy field? But as I began to work with them, I quickly realized that crystals are far from ordinary. Each one carries its own unique vibration, a sort of energetic fingerprint that can interact with and influence our own energy fields.

You see, everything in the universe is made up of energy vibrating at different frequencies. Crystals, formed over millions of years deep within the Earth, have some of the most stable and consistent vibrations in the natural world. When we bring these stable vibrations into contact with our own energy fields, which can often be chaotic or imbalanced, something magical happens. The crystals can help to realign and harmonize our energy, much like a tuning fork helps to bring a musical instrument back into tune.

Selecting the Right Crystals for Aura Healing

Now, you might be wondering, "With so many crystals out there, how do I know which ones to use for my aura?" It's a great question, and the answer lies in understanding both the properties of different crystals and the specific needs of your own energy field.

Let's start with some of the most commonly used crystals for aura healing:

Clear Quartz: Often called the "master healer," clear quartz is excellent for overall aura cleansing and amplification. It can help to clear blockages and boost the energy of other crystals.

Amethyst: This beautiful purple stone is wonderful for spiritual protection and cleansing. It can help to seal any tears in your aura and promote spiritual growth.

Rose Quartz: Known as the stone of love, rose quartz is perfect for healing emotional wounds in your aura. It promotes self-love and can help to soothe a damaged heart chakra.

Citrine: This sunny yellow crystal is fantastic for boosting confidence and personal power. It can help to strengthen a weak solar plexus chakra and bring more vitality to your aura.

Black Tourmaline: One of the most powerful protective stones, black tourmaline is excellent for grounding and shielding your aura from negative energies.

Selenite: This pure white crystal is like liquid light for your aura. It can help to cleanse and purify your energy field, washing away any stagnant or negative energies.

When selecting crystals, trust your intuition. You might find yourself drawn to a particular stone, even if you're not sure why.

This is often your energy field recognizing what it needs. Don't be afraid to explore and experiment with different crystals to see which ones resonate with you the most.

Understanding Your Aura's Needs

Before we dive into specific techniques for using crystals, it's important to take a moment to assess your aura's current state. Remember, your aura is a reflection of your physical, emotional, and spiritual well-being. Are you feeling drained or depleted? Your aura might need some energetic boosting. Feeling overwhelmed by others' emotions? Your aura might need some protection and strengthening. Struggling with old emotional wounds? Your aura might need some gentle, loving healing.

Take a few deep breaths and tune into your body and emotions. What areas feel like they need attention? This awareness will guide you in choosing the right crystals and techniques for your unique needs.

Techniques for Crystal Aura Healing

Now that we've covered the basics, let's explore some practical techniques for using crystals to heal and strengthen your aura.

Aura Scanning with Crystals

This technique can help you become more aware of your aura's condition and identify areas that need healing. Here's how to do it:

1. Choose a crystal that you're drawn to, preferably one with a point.

2. Lie down in a comfortable position and take a few deep breaths to center yourself.

3. Hold the crystal about 6 inches above your body, starting at your feet.

4. Slowly move the crystal up your body, paying attention to any sensations you feel. The crystal might feel heavier, lighter, or start to vibrate in certain areas.

5. Make note of these areas – they often correspond to parts of your aura that need attention.

Crystal Aura Cleansing

This technique is great for removing any stagnant or negative energy from your aura:

1. Select a cleansing crystal like clear quartz or selenite.

2. Stand with your feet shoulder-width apart and hold the crystal in your dominant hand.

3. Starting at your feet, make sweeping motions up your body with the crystal, imagining it collecting any unwanted energy.

4. When you reach your head, flick the crystal away from your body as if you're flinging off the negative energy.

5. Repeat this process 3-7 times, or until you feel a sense of lightness and clarity.

Aura Patching with Crystals

For repairing tears or weak spots in your aura:

1. Use your intuition or the aura scanning technique to identify areas that need repair.

2. Choose a crystal that corresponds to the area or issue you're working on. For example, rose quartz for emotional healing or amethyst for spiritual protection.

3. Lie down and place the crystal directly on the area of your body that corresponds to the weakened part of your aura.

4. Visualize the crystal's energy flowing into your aura, sealing any tears and strengthening the energy field.

5. Leave the crystal in place for 15-20 minutes, or until you feel a shift in the energy.

Crystal Aura Charging

To boost and energize your entire aura:

1. Select 7 crystals, one for each chakra. You can use clear quartz for all if you don't have a full set.

2. Lie down and place each crystal on its corresponding chakra point.

3. Close your eyes and visualize each crystal glowing with vibrant light, infusing your aura with its energy.

4. Stay in this position for 15-30 minutes, allowing the crystals to recharge your energy field.

Crystal Grids for Aura Protection and Healing

Crystal grids are a powerful way to combine the energies of multiple stones for a specific purpose. Here's a simple grid you can create for aura protection and healing:

1. On a clean surface, place a clear quartz point in the center, pointing away from you.

2. Around this central stone, arrange six other crystals in a hexagonal shape. You might use amethyst, rose quartz, citrine, black tourmaline, selenite, and fluorite.

3. Connect the stones by drawing lines between them with your finger, activating the grid.

4. Set your intention for aura healing and protection, then sit near the grid for meditation or leave it in your space to continually work on your energy field.

Carrying Crystals for Ongoing Aura Support

While dedicated healing sessions are wonderful, you can also benefit from the continuous support of crystals throughout your day. Here are some ways to keep crystal energy close:

Wear crystal jewelry: This is a beautiful and practical way to keep healing vibrations close to your aura. Choose pieces that contain stones aligned with your current needs.

Carry pocket stones: Select a few small, tumbled stones to carry in your pocket or purse. You can hold them when you need a quick energy boost or protection.

Create a crystal elixir: Place a clean, safe-for-water crystal in a glass of water overnight (research which crystals are safe for this method). In the morning, remove the crystal and drink the water to infuse your body and aura with crystal energy.

Cleansing and Charging Your Crystals

Remember, crystals absorb and transmute energy, so it's important to cleanse them regularly, especially when using them for aura healing. Here are some methods:

Moonlight: Leave your crystals outside or on a windowsill during a full moon.

Sunlight: Some crystals benefit from a few hours in the sun, but be careful as some can fade (like amethyst).

Smudging: Pass your crystals through the smoke of sage, palo santo, or incense.

Sound: Use a singing bowl or bell, allowing the vibrations to cleanse the crystals.

Visualization: Hold the crystals and visualize pure, white light flowing through them, clearing away any absorbed energies.

Developing Your Crystal Intuition

As you work more with crystals, you'll likely find that your intuition around them grows stronger. You might start to feel the energy of different stones more clearly or receive insights about which crystals you need at different times. Trust this growing awareness – it's a sign that you're becoming more attuned to the subtle energies around you.

I remember when I first started working with crystals, I often second-guessed myself. But over time, I learned to trust the gentle nudges I felt towards certain stones. Now, I can often sense exactly which crystal I need for a particular situation, and the results never cease to amaze me.

Combining Crystal Healing with Other Aura Repair Techniques

While crystals are powerful tools on their own, they can also enhance other aura healing techniques we've explored in previous chapters. For example:

During meditation: Hold a crystal or place it on your third eye to deepen your practice and enhance visualization.

In conjunction with color therapy: Use crystals that correspond to the colors you're working with to amplify the effects.

With sound healing: Place crystals around you during sound baths or when using singing bowls to create a harmonious energy field.

During energy work: Hold crystals or place them on the body during Reiki or other energy healing sessions to boost the effects.

When to Seek Professional Help

While working with crystals for aura healing can be incredibly beneficial, it's important to remember that they are a complementary tool, not a replacement for professional medical or psychological care. If you're dealing with serious physical or emotional issues, please consult with appropriate healthcare providers.

That being said, many energy healers and holistic practitioners are well-versed in crystal healing and can offer guided sessions that may be more potent than self-treatment. Consider seeking out a reputable crystal healer if you feel you need additional support or want to deepen your practice.

Embracing the Journey of Crystal Aura Healing

As we conclude this chapter, I want to encourage you to approach crystal healing with an open heart and mind. The journey of working with crystals is often one of self-discovery and increasing awareness of the energetic world around us. Each person's experience with crystals is unique, so don't be discouraged if your journey looks different from someone else's.

Remember, the most important factors in crystal healing are your intention and your willingness to work with the energies. The crystals are there to support and amplify your own healing abilities. Trust in the process, and trust in yourself.

As you continue to explore the world of crystal healing for your aura, you may find that it opens doors to new perceptions and experiences. You might start to sense energies more clearly, or develop a deeper understanding of your own energy field. Embrace these changes and allow them to guide you on your path of growth and healing.

In our next chapter, we'll explore another powerful modality for aura healing: color therapy and light work. You'll discover how to use the vibrant energies of color and light to further enhance and balance your aura. But for now, I encourage you to take some time to practice the crystal healing techniques we've discussed. Notice how different crystals affect your energy, and start building your own healing toolkit.

Remember, healing your aura is a journey, not a destination. Each step you take, each crystal you work with, is part of your unique path towards energetic balance and wellbeing. Trust the process, listen to your intuition, and most importantly, enjoy the beautiful, transformative power of crystal healing.

Chapter 13 - Color Therapy and Light Work

As we journey deeper into the realm of aura healing, we encounter two powerful tools that have been used for centuries to restore balance and vitality to our energy fields: color therapy and light work. In this chapter, we'll explore how these fascinating modalities can be harnessed to strengthen and heal your aura, providing you with practical techniques to incorporate into your daily life.

The Power of Color

Color is all around us, influencing our moods, emotions, and even our physical well-being. But have you ever stopped to consider how deeply color affects your energy field? As we've discussed in earlier chapters, the aura itself is often perceived as a rainbow of colors, each hue carrying its own unique vibration and meaning. By understanding and working with these colors, we can tap into a potent source of healing energy.

I remember the first time I truly understood the impact of color on my own energy. I was going through a particularly stressful period in my life, and a friend suggested I try wearing more blue. Skeptical but willing to try anything, I began incorporating more blue into my wardrobe. To my surprise, I found myself feeling calmer and more centered within just a few days. This personal experience led me down the path of exploring color therapy, and I'm excited to share what I've learned with you.

Understanding Chromotherapy

Chromotherapy, also known as color therapy, is the practice of using color and light to balance the body's energy centers or chakras. This ancient healing technique has roots in Egyptian, Greek, and Chinese cultures, where it was believed that different colors could promote healing and balance in the body and mind.

In the context of aura healing, chromotherapy can be a powerful tool for addressing imbalances and strengthening your energy field. Each color corresponds to a specific vibration and can be used to target particular issues or enhance certain qualities in your aura.

The Color Spectrum and Your Aura

Let's take a closer look at how different colors can affect your aura:

Red: Associated with the root chakra, red energy can help ground you and boost your physical vitality. If you're feeling lethargic or disconnected from your body, incorporating red into your aura healing practice can be beneficial.

Orange: Linked to the sacral chakra, orange energy stimulates creativity and emotional balance. It can be particularly helpful if you're feeling stuck or emotionally blocked.

Yellow: Connected to the solar plexus chakra, yellow energy promotes mental clarity and self-confidence. If you're struggling with self-doubt or mental fog, working with yellow can help clear and strengthen your aura.

Green: Associated with the heart chakra, green energy fosters healing, balance, and compassion. It's an excellent color to work with if you're recovering from emotional wounds or seeking to open your heart.

Blue: Linked to the throat chakra, blue energy enhances communication and self-expression. If you're having trouble speaking your truth or feeling heard, blue can help clear and strengthen this area of your aura.

Indigo: Connected to the third eye chakra, indigo energy promotes intuition and spiritual awareness. Working with this color can help you develop your psychic abilities and deepen your spiritual connection.

Violet: Associated with the crown chakra, violet energy connects you to higher consciousness and divine wisdom. It's an excellent color to work with if you're seeking spiritual growth or enlightenment.

Practical Color Therapy Techniques

Now that we understand the basics of how color affects our aura, let's explore some practical techniques you can use to harness the healing power of color:

Visualization: Close your eyes and imagine yourself surrounded by a particular color of light. Visualize this light penetrating your aura, cleansing and strengthening your energy field. You can focus on a single color that resonates with your current needs, or work your way through the entire spectrum for a complete aura "tune-up."

Colored Light Bathing: Use colored light bulbs or filters to bathe yourself in specific colors. You can create a dedicated space for this practice or simply replace some of the bulbs in your home with colored alternatives. Spend time each day basking in the colored light, allowing it to saturate your aura.

Color Breathing: This technique combines color visualization with breathwork. As you inhale, imagine drawing a specific color of light into your body and aura. As you exhale, visualize any negativity or stagnant energy leaving your body as gray or black smoke. This practice can be particularly effective for clearing and recharging your energy field.

Wearing Colors: As I mentioned earlier, the clothes we wear can have a significant impact on our energy. Try incorporating colors that correspond to the areas of your aura you want to strengthen into your wardrobe. You might be surprised at how quickly you notice a difference in your mood and energy levels.

Color Meditation: Create a meditation practice focused on a particular color. You might visualize yourself surrounded by that color, or focus on an object of that color as you meditate. This can help you attune to the specific vibration of the color and integrate its healing properties into your aura.

The Healing Power of Light

While color therapy focuses on specific hues, light work encompasses a broader spectrum of healing techniques that utilize various forms of light. Light is, after all, the source of all color, and working with light directly can be a powerful way to cleanse and strengthen your aura.

Sunlight Therapy

The sun is our most abundant and natural source of light, and spending time in sunlight can have a profound effect on your aura. Sunlight is rich in vitamin D, which is essential for physical health, but it also carries a high vibrational energy that can help cleanse and energize your aura.

To practice sunlight therapy, find a safe place to sit or lie in direct sunlight. Close your eyes and feel the warmth of the sun on your skin. Visualize the sunlight penetrating your aura, cleansing away any negativity and filling your energy field with vibrant, golden light. Start with just a few minutes a day and gradually increase your exposure, always being mindful of sun safety.

I often recommend this practice to my clients who are feeling depleted or stuck. One client, Sarah, had been struggling with low energy and a feeling of heaviness in her aura. After incorporating daily sunlight therapy into her routine for just two weeks, she reported feeling significantly lighter and more energized. The key is consistency and mindfulness – approach this practice with intention, and you'll likely notice positive changes in your energy field.

Moonlight Bathing

Just as the sun offers powerful healing energy, so too does the moon. Moonlight carries a softer, more subtle energy that can be particularly beneficial for emotional and spiritual healing. Many people find that working with moonlight helps to balance their feminine energy and enhance their intuitive abilities.

To practice moonlight bathing, find a safe outdoor space where you can sit or lie under the light of the full moon. Allow the gentle lunar energy to wash over you, visualizing it cleansing and renewing your aura. This practice can be especially powerful during a full moon, but you can work with moonlight at any phase of the lunar cycle.

Crystal Light Therapy

Crystals have long been used in energy healing, and when combined with light, they can offer a potent form of aura therapy. Different crystals resonate with different colors and energies, allowing you to target specific areas of your aura for healing.

To practice crystal light therapy, choose a crystal that corresponds to the area of your aura you want to work on. For example, you might choose a piece of rose quartz for heart chakra healing, or amethyst for spiritual growth. Hold the crystal up to a light source, allowing the light to pass through it and project onto your body. Sit or lie in this light for 10-15 minutes, visualizing the crystal-infused light penetrating and healing your aura.

Light Box Therapy

Light boxes, typically used to treat seasonal affective disorder, can also be beneficial for aura healing. These devices emit a bright light that mimics natural sunlight, helping to boost mood and energy levels. While not specifically designed for aura work, many of my clients have found that regular use of a light box helps to strengthen and brighten their energy field, particularly during darker winter months.

To incorporate light box therapy into your aura healing practice, set up your light box according to the manufacturer's instructions. Sit in front of it for 20-30 minutes each day, preferably in the morning. As you bask in the light, visualize it cleansing and energizing your aura. You might even combine this with color therapy by imagining the light taking on different hues as it penetrates your energy field.

Candle Gazing

Candle gazing, or trataka, is an ancient yogic practice that can be adapted for aura healing. This technique involves focusing your gaze on a candle flame, which can help to clear your mind, improve concentration, and cleanse your aura.

To practice candle gazing, sit in a comfortable position in a darkened room with a lit candle placed at eye level about an arm's length away. Focus your gaze softly on the flame, allowing your eyes to relax. If your eyes start to water or feel strained, gently close them and visualize the flame in your mind's eye. Practice for 5-10 minutes, gradually increasing the duration as you become more comfortable with the technique.

As you gaze at the flame, imagine it burning away any negativity or stagnant energy in your aura. Visualize your energy field becoming clearer and brighter with each moment of focus. Many of my students have reported feeling a sense of mental clarity and energetic lightness after practicing candle gazing regularly.

Integrating Color Therapy and Light Work

While each of these techniques can be powerful on its own, the real magic happens when you begin to integrate color therapy and light work into a comprehensive aura healing practice. Here are a few ways you can combine these modalities:

Colored Light Meditation: Use colored light bulbs or filters in combination with meditation. For example, you might meditate in a room bathed in blue light to enhance communication and self-expression.

Crystal Sunlight Therapy: Place crystals in a sunny window and sit in the colorful light they cast. This combines the healing properties of sunlight, crystal energy, and color therapy.

Moonlight Color Visualization: During your moonlight bathing sessions, incorporate color visualization. You might imagine the moonlight taking on different hues as it cleanses and recharges your aura.

Chakra Light Work: Create a practice that works through each chakra using corresponding colors and light sources. For example, you might use a red light or visualize red light for your root chakra, then move up through the spectrum to violet for your crown chakra.

Creating Your Personal Color and Light Healing Ritual

As with any healing practice, the key to success with color therapy and light work is consistency and personalization. I encourage you to experiment with the techniques we've discussed and create a ritual that resonates with you. Here's a sample ritual to get you started:

1. Begin your day with 10 minutes of sunlight therapy, visualizing golden light cleansing and energizing your aura.

2. Choose a color that corresponds to your intentions for the day. Wear something in that color or carry a crystal of that hue.

3. During your lunch break, practice color breathing for 5 minutes, focusing on the color you chose for the day.

4. In the evening, spend 15 minutes in meditation, visualizing yourself surrounded by healing light in various colors.

5. Before bed, practice 5 minutes of candle gazing to clear your mind and aura.

Remember, this is just a suggestion. Feel free to adapt and modify based on your schedule, preferences, and specific healing needs.

Cautions and Considerations

While color therapy and light work are generally safe practices, there are a few considerations to keep in mind:

Photosensitivity: Some individuals may be sensitive to certain types of light. If you experience headaches, eye strain, or other discomfort, reduce the intensity or duration of your light therapy sessions.

Sun Safety: When practicing sunlight therapy, always follow sun safety guidelines to protect your skin from damage.

Epilepsy: If you have epilepsy or are prone to seizures, consult with a healthcare professional before engaging in any practices involving flashing or intense lights.

Emotional Responses: Working with color and light can sometimes bring up strong emotions or memories. Be gentle with yourself and seek support if needed.

Conclusion

Color therapy and light work offer a vibrant and powerful approach to aura healing. By harnessing the energy of different colors and light sources, you can cleanse, strengthen, and balance your energy field, leading to greater overall well-being. As you incorporate these techniques into your daily life, pay attention to how different colors and types of light affect you. Your intuition is your best guide in this colorful journey of healing and self-discovery.

As we move forward, we'll explore another fascinating aspect of energy healing: the use of sound and vibration to harmonize and heal the aura. The world of energy is full of wonders, and I'm excited to continue this journey with you. Remember, your aura is as unique as you are – honor it, nurture it, and watch as it blossoms in radiant health and vitality.

Chapter 14 - Sound and Vibrational Healing for Your Energy Field

In the vast symphony of the universe, everything vibrates at its own unique frequency. From the tiniest subatomic particles to the grandest celestial bodies, all matter is in constant motion, creating an intricate dance of energy. Your aura, the subtle energy field that surrounds and interpenetrates your physical body, is no exception to this universal principle. It, too, resonates with its own specific vibrations, reflecting your physical, emotional, and spiritual state.

As we delve into the fascinating world of sound and vibrational healing for your energy field, we'll explore how these ancient and powerful techniques can be used to harmonize, balance, and rejuvenate your aura. By the end of this chapter, you'll have a deep understanding of how sound affects your energy field and practical tools to incorporate sound healing into your daily life.

The Science of Sound and Energy

Before we dive into specific healing techniques, it's important to understand the fundamental relationship between sound and energy. Sound is, at its core, a form of energy transmitted through vibrations. When you hear a sound, what you're actually perceiving are pressure waves traveling through the air, causing your eardrums to vibrate.

But sound isn't just limited to what we can hear. The universe is filled with vibrations beyond our auditory range, from the low rumbles of earthquakes to the high-frequency oscillations of light.

All of these vibrations interact with matter, including the subtle energy of your aura.

In the realm of quantum physics, we've discovered that everything in the universe is essentially energy vibrating at different frequencies. This includes your thoughts, emotions, and even your physical body. When we use sound for healing, we're essentially using one form of vibrational energy to influence another.

The concept of resonance is crucial to understanding how sound healing works. Resonance occurs when the frequency of one object matches the natural frequency of another, causing the second object to vibrate in sympathy. This principle is at the heart of how sound can affect your aura and, by extension, your overall well-being.

Understanding Your Aura's Frequency

Your aura, like everything else in the universe, has its own unique vibrational signature. This signature is a complex interplay of different frequencies, each corresponding to various aspects of your being – physical, emotional, mental, and spiritual.

When you're in good health and your energy is balanced, your aura vibrates in harmony with your true nature. However, stress, illness, emotional trauma, and other disruptive factors can cause discordance in your energy field. This is where sound healing comes in.

By introducing specific frequencies through sound, we can help bring your aura back into balance. It's like tuning a musical instrument – we're adjusting the vibrations of your energy field to restore harmony and optimal functioning.

The Healing Power of Music

Music has been used for healing and spiritual purposes for thousands of years across cultures worldwide. There's a reason why certain melodies can bring tears to your eyes, while others make you want to get up and dance. Music has a profound effect on our emotions, our physiology, and yes, our energy field.

When you listen to music that resonates with you, you might notice a shift in your mood or energy level. This is because the vibrations of the music are interacting with your aura, potentially helping to balance and harmonize your energy.

Different types of music can have varying effects on your aura:

Classical music, especially compositions by Mozart and Bach, has been found to have a harmonizing effect on the energy field. The complex structures and mathematical precision of these pieces can help bring order to a chaotic aura.

Native American flute music, with its soulful, earthy tones, can be particularly effective for grounding and connecting with the root chakra.

Tibetan singing bowl music creates rich, multi-layered tones that can help balance and align all the chakras, promoting overall aura health.

Ambient or new age music, with its flowing, ethereal quality, can help expand and cleanse the aura, promoting a sense of spaciousness and peace.

When using music for aura healing, I encourage you to trust your intuition. The music that feels most healing to you is likely what your energy field needs at that moment. Set aside time each day to listen mindfully to music, allowing the vibrations to wash over and through you, imagining them cleansing and balancing your aura.

The Power of Your Own Voice

While listening to music can be incredibly healing, don't underestimate the power of your own voice as a tool for aura healing. Your voice is uniquely attuned to your own energy field, making it a potent instrument for self-healing.

Toning is a simple yet powerful technique you can use. To practice toning, simply take a deep breath and, on the exhale, make a sustained vowel sound like "ah," "oh," or "om." As you make the sound, visualize it resonating throughout your body and aura, clearing away any stagnant or discordant energy.

Each vowel sound is associated with different areas of the body and aspects of the aura:

"Ah" resonates with the heart center and can help open and balance the heart chakra.

"Oh" connects with the solar plexus, aiding in confidence and personal power.

"Ee" vibrates with the third eye chakra, enhancing intuition and clarity.

"Oo" relates to the throat chakra, supporting clear communication and self-expression.

"Om," considered the primordial sound in many Eastern traditions, is said to vibrate with the crown chakra and can help connect you with higher consciousness.

Experiment with these sounds and notice how they make you feel. You might find that certain tones resonate more strongly with you or seem to have a more noticeable effect on your energy.

Mantras and Chanting

Mantras, sacred sounds or phrases repeated in meditation, have been used for thousands of years in various spiritual traditions to alter consciousness and heal the subtle body. When you chant a mantra, you're not just saying words – you're creating a specific vibration that interacts with your energy field.

One of the most well-known mantras is the Sanskrit "Om Mani Padme Hum," which is said to contain the essence of all Buddhist teachings. Each syllable of this mantra is associated with purifying different aspects of your being:

"Om" purifies the body
"Ma" purifies the speech
"Ni" purifies the mind
"Pad" purifies the qualities
"Me" purifies the method
"Hum" purifies the wisdom

As you chant this or any other mantra, visualize its vibrations permeating your aura, cleansing and balancing your energy field. The repetitive nature of mantra chanting can also help quiet the mind and induce a meditative state, further supporting aura healing.

Tuning Forks for Precision Healing

Tuning forks offer a precise way to introduce specific frequencies into your energy field. These simple tools, originally used to tune musical instruments, have become popular in sound healing due to their ability to produce pure, clear tones.

Different tuning forks are calibrated to different frequencies, each associated with specific healing properties. For example:

The 128 Hz fork is often used for grounding and connecting with Earth energy.

The 432 Hz fork is said to resonate with the natural frequency of the universe and can help bring your energy into harmony with nature.

The 528 Hz fork, sometimes called the "love frequency," is associated with transformation and miracles.

To use a tuning fork for aura healing, strike it gently and then hold it near different parts of your body, allowing the vibrations to penetrate your energy field. You can also move the fork in circles around your body to help clear and balance your aura.

Some practitioners use sets of tuning forks tuned to the frequencies of the planets, chakras, or other significant vibrations. These can be used in various patterns to create "sonic acupuncture," targeting specific points in the energy field.

Singing Bowls: Ancient Tools for Modern Healing

Singing bowls, whether Tibetan metal bowls or crystal quartz bowls, produce complex, multi-layered tones that can have a profound effect on your aura. The rich harmonics created by these instruments seem to envelop you in sound, facilitating a deep state of relaxation and meditation.

To use a singing bowl for aura healing, you can either play it yourself or listen to recordings. If you're using the bowl yourself, try this simple exercise:

Hold the bowl in your non-dominant hand, or place it on a cushion in front of you.

Using a mallet, gently strike the rim of the bowl to produce a clear, ringing tone.

As the sound fades, run the mallet around the rim of the bowl to create a sustained "singing" tone.

Close your eyes and visualize the sound waves moving through your aura, clearing away any stuck or stagnant energy and restoring balance.

Different sized bowls produce different tones, which can be used to target specific chakras or areas of the aura. Larger bowls with deeper tones are often used for grounding and working with the lower chakras, while smaller bowls with higher pitches can help clear and balance the upper chakras.

Binaural Beats: Modern Technology for Brainwave Entrainment

Binaural beats represent a more modern approach to sound healing. This technology uses slightly different frequencies played in each ear to create a perceived beat at the difference between the two frequencies. For example, if a 400 Hz tone is played in your left ear and a 410 Hz tone in your right, your brain perceives a 10 Hz beat.

The fascinating aspect of binaural beats is that they can entrain your brainwaves to match the perceived beat frequency. Different brainwave states are associated with different states of consciousness:

Delta waves (0.5-4 Hz) are linked to deep sleep and healing.

Theta waves (4-8 Hz) are associated with deep relaxation and meditation.

Alpha waves (8-14 Hz) promote relaxation and creativity.

Beta waves (14-30 Hz) are our normal waking state, associated with focused attention.

Gamma waves (30-100 Hz) are linked to higher cognitive function and spiritual experiences.

By using binaural beats, you can guide your brain into specific states that support healing and balance in your aura. For example, theta binaural beats can help you access a deep meditative state, facilitating energy healing and chakra balancing.

To use binaural beats effectively, you'll need to listen with stereo headphones. Many apps and online resources offer binaural beat tracks for various purposes. As with all healing modalities, pay attention to how you feel and trust your intuition about what works best for you.

Gongs: Cosmic Sounds for Deep Healing

The gong is one of the most powerful instruments for sound healing, capable of producing an incredible range of tones and overtones. A skilled gong player can create a "sound bath" that seems to transport you to other realms of consciousness.

The complex vibrations produced by a gong can help break up stagnant energy in your aura, release blockages, and promote a sense of expansion and connection with the universe. Many people report profound experiences during gong meditations, including visions, emotional releases, and deep insights.

If you have the opportunity to experience a live gong meditation, I highly recommend it. The physical presence of the sound waves can be felt throughout your body and aura in a way that recordings can't fully replicate. However, even recorded gong meditations can be powerfully effective for aura healing.

When participating in a gong meditation, whether live or recorded, try this visualization:

Imagine your aura as a sphere of light surrounding your body.

As the gong sounds begin, visualize the sound waves moving through your aura like ripples on a pond.

See these ripples clearing away any dark or cloudy areas in your energy field, leaving your aura bright, clear, and vibrant.

Allow yourself to fully immerse in the experience, letting go of any expectations and simply being present with the sound.

Nature Sounds for Aura Healing

In our modern world, we're often disconnected from the healing sounds of nature. Yet, natural soundscapes can be incredibly effective for balancing and healing the aura. The sounds of forests, oceans, rainstorms, and birdsong all carry specific vibrations that can help harmonize your energy field.

Ocean waves, with their rhythmic ebb and flow, can help balance the emotional body and promote a sense of calm and expansiveness in your aura.

Rainforest sounds, with their rich tapestry of bird calls, insect chirps, and rustling leaves, can help clear mental chatter and promote a sense of connection with the natural world.

Thunderstorms, with the deep rumble of thunder and the patter of rain, can be powerfully cleansing for the aura, helping to release pent-up emotions and stagnant energy.

Birdsong, particularly in the early morning, can help awaken and enliven your energy field, promoting a sense of joy and possibility.

Try incorporating nature sounds into your daily routine. You might listen to ocean waves as you fall asleep, use rainforest sounds as background during your workday, or take a walk in nature and consciously tune in to the sounds around you.

Incorporating Sound Healing into Your Daily Life

Now that we've explored various sound healing techniques, you might be wondering how to incorporate them into your daily life. Here are some suggestions:

Start your day with a sound healing session. This could be as simple as chanting a mantra, listening to singing bowl music as you meditate, or using tuning forks to balance your energy before you begin your day.

Use music intentionally throughout your day. Choose music that supports the energy you want to cultivate. For example, you might listen to grounding earth drumming while cooking, uplifting classical music while working, or peaceful ambient sounds while winding down in the evening.

Take sound breaks. Instead of scrolling through your phone during breaks, try a short toning session or listen to a nature sound recording to reset your energy.

End your day with soothing sounds. Use gentle music, singing bowls, or nature sounds to help you transition into sleep, allowing the healing vibrations to work on your aura as you rest.

Attend sound healing events. Many communities offer group sound baths or gong meditations. These can be powerful experiences and also connect you with others interested in energy healing.

Create a personal sound healing toolkit. This might include a singing bowl, some tuning forks, a selection of healing music, and perhaps a small drum or rattle.

Remember, consistency is key in any healing practice. Even a few minutes of intentional sound healing each day can have a significant impact on your aura over time.

Combining Sound Healing with Other Modalities

While sound healing is powerful on its own, it can also be effectively combined with other healing modalities to enhance its effects on your aura. Here are some combinations to explore:

Sound and Crystal Healing: Place crystals on or around your body during sound healing sessions. The vibrations of the sound can amplify the healing properties of the crystals.

Sound and Color Therapy: Visualize specific colors in your aura as you work with different sounds. For example, you might visualize golden light filling your aura as you listen to Tibetan singing bowls.

Sound and Aromatherapy: Certain essential oils can help open you to the healing effects of sound. Try using lavender for relaxation, peppermint for clarity, or frankincense for spiritual connection during your sound healing sessions.

Sound and Movement: Gentle movement practices like tai chi or qigong can be enhanced by incorporating sound. Try toning or chanting as you move through your practice.

Sound and Breathwork: Conscious breathing combined with sound can be a powerful way to move energy through your aura. Try inhaling deeply and exhaling with a long "om" sound.

As with all healing practices, trust your intuition and pay attention to what feels right for you. Your aura is unique, and you may find that certain combinations work particularly well for your energy field.

Precautions and Considerations

While sound healing is generally safe for most people, there are a few precautions to keep in mind:

Volume: Always use a comfortable volume, especially when using headphones. Extremely loud sounds can be damaging to both your physical hearing and your subtle energy field.

Emotional Responses: Sound healing can sometimes trigger emotional releases. This is normal and often part of the healing process, but be gentle with yourself and seek support if needed.

Pregnancy: If you're pregnant, consult with your healthcare provider before engaging in intense sound healing practices, particularly those involving low frequencies or physical vibrations.

Medical Conditions: If you have a seizure disorder or other neurological condition, check with your doctor before using binaural beats or other brainwave entrainment technologies.

Overwhelm: If you feel overwhelmed or uncomfortable during a sound healing session, it's okay to take a break or stop. Trust your body's signals.

Quality of Sound: Use high-quality recordings and instruments when possible. Poor quality sounds or harsh, jarring noises can potentially create dissonance in your energy field.

As we conclude this exploration of sound and vibrational healing for your aura, I hope you're feeling inspired to incorporate these practices into your life. Remember, your voice, your breath, and even your heartbeat are all forms of sound healing available to you at any moment.

The universe is a grand symphony, and you are both an instrument and a conductor in this cosmic orchestra. By working consciously with sound, you have the power to tune your personal energy field, harmonizing with the vibrations of health, balance, and wellbeing.

In our next chapter, we'll explore another crucial aspect of aura health: protective practices for shielding your energy field. But for now, I encourage you to sit for a moment in silence, tuning in to the subtle sounds around and within you. In this awareness, you're already beginning to heal and balance your aura through the power of sound.

Chapter 15 - Protective Practices: Shielding Your Aura

As we journey through life, our energy fields are constantly interacting with the world around us. While these interactions can be enriching and enlightening, they can also leave us vulnerable to negative influences and energy drain. This is where protective practices come into play, offering us the tools to shield our auras and maintain our energetic integrity.

In this chapter, we'll explore essential techniques for creating energetic boundaries and shields to protect your aura from external influences and energy drain. By mastering these practices, you'll be better equipped to navigate the energetic landscape of your daily life, maintaining your vitality and well-being in the face of various challenges.

Understanding the Need for Aura Protection

Before we dive into specific techniques, it's important to understand why protecting your aura is so crucial. Think of your aura as a delicate, yet powerful, energy field that surrounds and interpenetrates your physical body. This field is sensitive to the energies around you, both positive and negative.

In my years of working with clients, I've often encountered individuals who feel drained after spending time in crowded places or with certain people. They describe feeling "not quite themselves" or experiencing unexplained mood shifts. These are classic signs of an unprotected aura absorbing external energies.

Your aura acts as a filter and a buffer between you and the world. When it's strong and well-protected, you're better able to maintain your emotional balance, mental clarity, and overall sense of well-being. However, when your aura is weak or unshielded, you become more susceptible to:

1. Energy vampires: People who, consciously or unconsciously, drain your energy.

2. Negative emotions from others: Absorbing the stress, anger, or sadness of those around you.

3. Environmental stressors: Such as electromagnetic fields or the chaotic energy of busy urban areas.

4. Psychic attacks: Intentional or unintentional negative energy directed at you by others.

By implementing protective practices, you create a resilient energetic barrier that allows you to engage with the world while maintaining your energetic integrity.

The Visualization Shield Technique

One of the most fundamental and versatile techniques for aura protection is the visualization shield. This method harnesses the power of your imagination to create a protective barrier around your energy field.

To begin, find a quiet place where you won't be disturbed. Close your eyes and take a few deep, calming breaths. As you relax, imagine a bright, warm light emanating from your heart center. This light represents your pure, vital energy.

Now, visualize this light expanding outward, enveloping your entire body. As it grows, see it forming a transparent, bubble-like shield around you. This shield can be any color that feels protective and comforting to you. Some people prefer a golden light, while others might choose a cool blue or a vibrant white.

Imagine this shield as a semi-permeable membrane. It allows positive energy to flow freely in and out, but it repels and deflects any negative or harmful energies. See it as strong, flexible, and resilient – able to withstand any energetic assaults while remaining adaptable to your needs.

Take a moment to feel the safety and security this shield provides. Know that you can call upon this protective barrier whenever you need it, whether you're entering a crowded space, preparing for a challenging interaction, or simply going about your day.

I often recommend that my clients practice this visualization first thing in the morning and last thing at night. By making it a regular part of your routine, you'll find it becomes second nature to maintain this protective shield throughout your day.

Grounding for Aura Protection

While shielding is crucial for protection, it's equally important to stay grounded. Grounding helps anchor your energy, preventing you from becoming too "spacey" or disconnected when working with protective practices.

One effective grounding technique is the "Tree Root" visualization. Stand with your feet shoulder-width apart and imagine your legs transforming into strong, sturdy tree roots. See these roots growing down from the soles of your feet, penetrating deep into the earth.

As you breathe in, visualize drawing up earth energy through these roots, feeling it fill your body with stable, grounding energy. As you exhale, release any excess or negative energy back into the earth, where it can be neutralized and transformed.

This grounding practice not only helps protect your aura but also provides a constant source of revitalizing earth energy. It's particularly useful when you're feeling overwhelmed or unbalanced.

The Power of Intention in Aura Protection

Never underestimate the power of your intention when it comes to protecting your aura. Your thoughts and beliefs play a significant role in shaping your energy field.

Start each day by setting a clear intention for your energetic protection. You might say something like, "I intend for my energy field to be strong, protected, and impermeable to negative influences." Repeat this intention throughout the day, especially when entering situations where you might feel energetically vulnerable.

I once worked with a client, Sarah, who was struggling with a particularly toxic work environment. She felt drained and demoralized every time she entered her office. We worked together to create a personalized intention for her aura protection. Each morning before work, she would affirm: "My aura is a fortress of light. I am protected from negative energies, and only positivity can enter my space."

Within weeks, Sarah reported feeling more resilient and less affected by the negativity around her. While her work environment hadn't changed, her ability to protect herself energetically had dramatically improved.

Creating Energetic Boundaries

In addition to shielding and grounding, it's essential to establish clear energetic boundaries. This involves being mindful of how you interact with others on an energetic level and learning to say "no" to energy-draining situations or relationships.

Start by becoming more aware of how different people and environments affect your energy. Do you feel uplifted and energized after spending time with certain friends? Do you feel drained and depleted after interacting with others? This awareness is the first step in creating healthy energetic boundaries.

Once you've identified energy-draining situations or relationships, practice setting firm but compassionate boundaries. This might involve limiting time spent with certain individuals, avoiding gossip or negative conversations, or excusing yourself from situations that feel energetically overwhelming.

Remember, setting boundaries is not about shutting people out, but about preserving your energy so you can show up fully in your life and relationships. It's an act of self-care that ultimately benefits not just you, but those around you as well.

The Cord-Cutting Ritual

Sometimes, despite our best efforts at protection, we may find ourselves energetically entangled with others in ways that drain our energy. This is where the cord-cutting ritual can be incredibly powerful.

Energetic cords are etheric connections that form between people, often in close relationships. While some cords can be positive and nurturing, others can be draining or even toxic. The cord-cutting ritual helps sever these unhealthy connections.

To perform a cord-cutting ritual, find a quiet space where you won't be disturbed. Close your eyes and take a few deep breaths to center yourself. Visualize the person with whom you feel you have an unhealthy energetic connection.

See or sense the cords connecting you to this person. These cords might appear as ropes, tubes, or strings of light. Now, imagine a pair of golden scissors in your hand. With intention and compassion, visualize yourself cutting these cords.

As you cut each cord, affirm: "I release this connection with love and compassion. I reclaim my energy and set us both free." Visualize the cut cords dissolving into light, returning any energy that belongs to you and releasing any that doesn't.

After cutting the cords, imagine your aura being filled with golden light, healing and sealing any places where the cords were attached. This ritual can be deeply liberating and is an important tool in maintaining strong aura protection.

Using Crystals for Aura Protection

Crystals can be powerful allies in protecting your aura. Different crystals have unique protective properties, and incorporating them into your daily life can significantly enhance your aura's resilience.

Some crystals particularly effective for aura protection include:

1. Black Tourmaline: Known for its grounding properties and ability to repel negative energy.

2. Amethyst: Helps create a protective shield around your aura and enhances spiritual awareness.

3. Selenite: Cleanses and charges the aura, creating a protective light barrier.

4. Hematite: Offers strong grounding energy and deflects negative influences.

5. Clear Quartz: Amplifies your intentions and can be programmed for specific protective purposes.

To use these crystals for aura protection, you can carry them with you, wear them as jewelry, or place them around your living and working spaces. You can also use them during meditation, holding them while visualizing your protective shield.

I often recommend that my clients create a "protection grid" in their homes using these crystals. Place a piece of Black Tourmaline in each corner of your home, with a central Clear Quartz to amplify the protective energy. This creates a stable, protective energy field throughout your living space.

The Protective Power of Salt

Salt has been used for centuries in various cultures for its purifying and protective properties. Incorporating salt into your aura protection practices can be a simple yet effective way to enhance your energetic defenses.

One method is to take a salt bath. Add a cup of sea salt or Himalayan pink salt to your bathwater and soak for at least 20 minutes. As you bathe, visualize the salt water cleansing your aura of any negative or stagnant energy. This practice is particularly beneficial after you've been in crowded or high-stress environments.

You can also create a protective salt spray for your aura. In a spray bottle, mix purified water with a tablespoon of sea salt. You can add a few drops of protective essential oils like lavender or frankincense if desired. Shake well and spray around your body, visualizing it creating a protective barrier around your aura.

For ongoing protection in your living space, consider placing small bowls of salt in the corners of your rooms. The salt absorbs negative energy and helps maintain a clean, protective atmosphere.

Aura Protection Through Breathwork

Your breath is a powerful tool for aura protection. Specific breathing techniques can help strengthen your energy field and create a protective buffer around you.

One effective technique is the "Protective Breath of Light." Begin by taking a deep breath in through your nose, imagining you're inhaling pure, white light. As you exhale through your mouth, visualize this light expanding to create a protective sphere around your entire body.

With each inhalation, see the light growing stronger and brighter. With each exhalation, feel your aura becoming more resilient and impenetrable to negative energies. Practice this for at least five minutes, or whenever you feel the need for immediate energetic protection.

Another powerful breathwork technique is alternate nostril breathing, or Nadi Shodhana in yoga practice. This balances the left and right hemispheres of your brain and harmonizes your energy field, making it more resilient to external influences.

To practice, use your right thumb to close your right nostril and inhale deeply through your left nostril. At the top of the inhalation, close your left nostril with your ring finger, release your thumb, and exhale through your right nostril. Inhale through the right nostril, then close it, exhale through the left, and repeat the cycle. Practice for 5-10 minutes to feel centered and protected.

The Role of Positive Affirmations in Aura Protection

The power of positive thinking extends to aura protection as well. Incorporating affirmations into your daily routine can significantly strengthen your aura's protective capabilities.

Create a set of personal affirmations that resonate with you. Some examples might include:

- "I am surrounded by a shield of divine light that protects me from all harm."

- "My aura is strong, resilient, and impenetrable to negative energies."

- "I choose what energies I allow into my space."

- "I am grounded, centered, and protected at all times."

Repeat these affirmations daily, particularly in the morning as you start your day and in the evening before you sleep. You can also use them throughout the day when you feel the need for extra protection.

The key is to really feel the truth of these statements as you say them. Visualize your aura growing stronger with each affirmation. Over time, these positive statements will become deeply ingrained in your subconscious, automatically reinforcing your aura's protective abilities.

Aura Protection in Challenging Environments

There are times when we find ourselves in environments that are particularly challenging from an energetic standpoint. This might be a crowded public space, a high-stress work environment, or even a gathering where there's conflict or tension.

In these situations, it's crucial to have quick and effective techniques for bolstering your aura's protection. One such technique is the "Zip-Up" method.

Stand up straight and imagine a zipper at your feet, running up the front of your body to the top of your head. Place your hands at your feet and, as you slowly stand up straight, visualize zipping up this energetic zipper. As you do this, affirm: "I am sealed and protected in my own energy."

This simple yet powerful technique creates an immediate energetic barrier, particularly useful when you're about to enter a challenging situation.

Another technique for instant protection is the "Bubble of Light" visualization. Imagine yourself surrounded by a bubble of pure, radiant light. See this bubble as flexible yet impenetrable, allowing only positive energy to pass through while deflecting any negative or harmful energies.

You can enhance this visualization by choosing a color for your bubble that feels particularly protective to you. Some people prefer a golden light for divine protection, while others might choose a deep blue for calm strength or a vibrant purple for spiritual shielding.

Maintaining Long-Term Aura Protection

While these techniques are powerful for immediate protection, maintaining long-term aura health requires consistent practice and awareness. Think of it as energetic hygiene – just as you shower and brush your teeth daily, your aura needs regular care and attention.

Develop a daily routine that incorporates some of the techniques we've discussed. This might include starting your day with a protective visualization, practicing grounding exercises throughout the day, and ending with a cleansing salt bath or meditation.

Regular energy cleansing is also crucial for maintaining strong aura protection. This can involve smudging with sage or palo santo, taking cleansing showers where you visualize negativity washing away, or using sound healing tools like singing bowls or tuning forks to clear your energy field.

It's also important to pay attention to your physical and emotional health. A strong, protected aura is supported by a healthy body and mind. Ensure you're getting enough rest, eating nourishing foods, staying hydrated, and engaging in regular physical exercise. Additionally, practices like journaling, counseling, or talking with trusted friends can help process emotions and prevent them from creating vulnerabilities in your aura.

The Spiritual Dimension of Aura Protection

For many, aura protection has a spiritual dimension. If this resonates with you, consider incorporating spiritual practices into your protective routine. This might involve prayer, calling upon spirit guides or guardian angels for protection, or working with specific deities associated with protection in your spiritual tradition.

You might create a protection altar in your home, with symbols, images, or objects that represent safety and divine protection to you. Spending time at this altar, meditating or simply sitting in quiet contemplation, can help reinforce your sense of spiritual protection.

Remember, the most powerful protection comes from a place of love, not fear. When you approach aura protection from a place of self-love and a desire for the highest good of all, you align yourself with the most potent protective forces in the universe.

Teaching Others About Aura Protection

As you become more adept at protecting your own aura, you may find yourself in a position to help others do the same. Whether you're a healing practitioner or simply someone who wants to support friends and loved ones, sharing these techniques can be a beautiful way to spread light and empowerment.

When teaching others about aura protection, it's important to emphasize that these practices are about personal empowerment, not fear. Encourage people to tune into their own intuition and find the methods that resonate most strongly with them.

You might organize a workshop or gathering where you guide people through various protection techniques. This can be a powerful way to create a community of support and shared knowledge around energetic self-care.

Conclusion: Embracing Your Energetic Sovereignty

As we conclude this chapter on protective practices for your aura, I want to emphasize that these techniques are not about isolation or disconnection from the world around you. Rather, they're tools for maintaining your energetic sovereignty – your right and ability to choose what energies you engage with and how you respond to the energetic environment around you.

By mastering these protective practices, you're not putting up walls, but rather creating a flexible, resilient energetic field that allows you to engage fully with life while maintaining your core essence. You're cultivating a strength that comes from within, a centered calm that can weather any energetic storm.

As you move forward, integrating these practices into your daily life, remember that aura protection is an ongoing journey. Be patient with yourself as you learn and grow. Celebrate the moments when you feel strong and centered, and be gentle with yourself during times when you feel more vulnerable.

Your aura is a beautiful, unique expression of your energy in this world. By protecting and nurturing it, you're honoring your true self and creating a foundation for profound healing and personal growth. As you strengthen your own protective abilities, you'll likely find that you naturally become a source of strength and protection for others as well, contributing to a more balanced and harmonious energetic environment for all.

In the next chapter, we'll explore how specific meditation and breathwork practices can further strengthen, expand, and balance your aura, providing you with even more tools for your energetic toolkit. But for now, take a moment to appreciate the protective power you hold within you. Your aura is your own personal shield of light – may it always shine brightly, keeping you safe and allowing your true essence to radiate into the world.

Chapter 16 - Aura Healing Through Meditation and Breathwork

Meeting Your Inner Shield

In the previous chapter I invited you to wrap your aura in protective light, to weave energetic fabrics so skillfully that heavy vibrations slid off like rain from a well-oiled cloak. Those shields are indispensable, yet even the most artfully constructed barrier is only as strong as the vitality inside it. A knight who dons armor but neglects his own health will not last long on the battlefield; in the same way, an aura that is merely walled off soon stagnates unless living currents continually refresh it from within. This is where meditation and breathwork step forward. They are not additions to the work we have done so far; they are its pulsing heart. By learning to guide your awareness and your breath, you learn to feed your auric field directly with the primal forces that sustain life itself.

I still remember the first time I felt the undeniable shimmer of my own aura during meditation. I was sitting on an old cork yoga mat in a studio that smelled faintly of lavender and cedar, following a teacher's calm instructions to "breathe through the skin." For an instant my logical mind protested—skin is not porous in that sense, I thought—but then I surrendered, drew in a slow breath, and imagined each pore opening like the minute petals of spring buds. A warm hum ignited around me, soft as down and unmistakably alive. In that moment I realized breath was more than a mechanical exchange of gases; it was a carrier wave of consciousness, capable of washing the energy field as surely as rain cleanses the earth.

That is the experience I want for you. Over the course of this chapter we will explore why meditation and breathwork are so critically linked to aura healing, how you can prepare yourself to practice, and a range of meditations—from simple to advanced—that directly replenish, mend, and expand your luminous field. We will navigate practical obstacles, look at real-world stories, and finally set the stage for our next exploration: how a well-nourished aura sets the tone for every relationship you enter.

Why Breath and Stillness Mend the Luminous Body

Modern science and ancient wisdom traditions often sound like distant relatives: they recognize each other around the dinner table yet still speak different dialects. When it comes to breath and meditation, however, their observations converge. Western physiology tells us that slow, diaphragmatic breathing activates the vagus nerve, nudging the nervous system into a parasympathetic, or "rest and digest," state. Heart rate variability improves, blood pressure normalizes, and inflammation markers drop. Meanwhile, MRI studies reveal that mindfulness meditation thickens gray matter in regions related to self-regulation and empathy. Translating that into the language of subtle energy, we can say that the nervous system's calmer frequencies permit the aura to untangle, brighten, and expand, while the enhanced gray-matter circuitry enables us to sense those energetic shifts with increasing clarity.

Eastern traditions speak of prana, qi, ruach, or pneuma—vital currents that enter primarily through breath, ride on intention, and suffuse every layer of the aura. Yogic texts describe the pranamaya kosha, the breath or life-force sheath, as the intermediary between the physical body and the subtler mental and bliss sheaths. When prana flows evenly, the aura is luminous and coherent. When it stagnates, dull patches or rips appear and, if ignored, eventually precipitate into emotional dissonance or physical illness. Thus, breath is not merely symbolic; it is the tangible handle by which we grasp invisible energetic levers.

Meditation amplifies this effect by steadying the mind, the very tool we use to direct prana. A distracted mind sprinkles vital energy haphazardly on worries, regrets, and imagined futures. A focused mind gathers that same energy and pours it deliberately into repair and growth. Imagine trying to paint a wall with a leaky bucket and a shaking hand; you would waste more paint than you applied. Meditation tightens the bucket, steadies the hand, and lets the color seep smoothly into every crack.

Setting the Stage: Environment, Posture, and Intention

Before we venture into specific practices, we need to arrange conditions so that your subtle body feels safe enough to open. Think of a flower that only unfolds when sunlight and moisture reach just the right balance. The environment where you meditate is that sunlight and moisture.

Choose a space where you can remain uninterrupted for the duration of your session. It does not have to be silent, but the sounds should be benign and predictable—rustling leaves, distant traffic, a neighbor's muffled footsteps. Sudden bursts of loud noise jerk the auric field, forcing it to contract defensively. If possible, air the room beforehand so that fresh oxygen feeds your breath. Some people like incense or essential oils; others prefer plain air. Trust your senses. If the aroma grounds you, by all means light the stick of sandalwood or add a drop of frankincense to a diffuser. If scents distract you, let the air remain unscented and pure.

Posture functions as architecture for energy flow. You can sit cross-legged on the floor, on a cushion, in a chair with feet flat, or even lie down if pain prevents sitting. The spine, however, must be long yet relaxed, like a young sapling swaying in the wind. A collapsed spine kinks energy channels; a rigid spine blocks natural micro-movements. I often imagine my vertebrae as a string of freshwater pearls, each one luminous and perfectly aligned, yet loose enough that they roll gently over each other as I breathe.

Once you are comfortable, frame a simple intention. Our earlier chapters taught you how intention colors energy; here the same principle applies. Perhaps you say quietly, "With each breath I invite healing light to mend and expand my aura." If spoken words feel awkward, let the intention form as a felt sense: the subtle, expectant hush you hold when someone you love is about to walk through the door. That expectancy, invisible yet palpable, is enough.

The Foundational Practice: Breath Awareness

Everything we do from this point branches out from a trunk called breath awareness. Before we sculpt and direct energy, we must know how it currently flows. A sculptor studies the grain of wood before chiseling.

Close your eyes. Allow your lips to part so the jaw muscles loosen. Inhale through the nose and let the air descend down the back of the throat, expanding the belly first, then the ribs, then the collarbones. Exhale gently, reversing the wave. For the first minute, do nothing else; simply observe the coolness of the incoming air, the warmth of the outgoing, the faint rub of fabric against your rib cage as it widens and contracts.

While you breathe, imagine your awareness dropping from the analyzing mind into the body. I like to picture small lanterns lighting up inside each cell; as they flicker to life, the inside of my skin becomes a star-studded sky. With each exhale, tension slides off those lanterns like wax, revealing brighter flames. You may feel tingles in your hands or a fuzzy halo around your head. These sensations are early signals that your aura is responding, fluffing up like a blanket shaken in sunlight.

If thoughts intrude—and they will—meet them the way you might greet a polite stranger while hurrying to an appointment. Nod, acknowledge, and move on. The breath is your appointment. Each time you choose breath over distraction, you strengthen the muscle that will later lift and weave luminous strands across tears in your energy field.

Practice for at least five minutes daily. Think of it as priming a pump; once groundwater flows steadily, you can irrigate any garden you choose, including the garden of your aura.

The Healing Wave: Expanding and Cleansing the Aura with Breath

After two weeks—or sooner if you feel ready—you can begin using your breath not merely to observe but actively to cleanse and repair. I call this the Healing Wave.

Begin with the same seated position and breath awareness. Now, on an inhale, visualize bright, shimmering light—perhaps golden, perhaps pure white—entering through the crown of your head. Let it course down the spinal column, pooling in the sacrum. Some feel it as a cool, sparkling waterfall; others, as a warm honey stream. Either image works, as long as it feels nourishing.

As you reach the top of the inhalation, hold for a gentle heartbeat or two, allowing the collected light to press outward. Then exhale, imagining the light radiating in every direction until it permeates and expands past the boundary of your physical body. Picture a soap bubble inflating around you, growing more iridescent with every breath cycle. On the out-breath, you also release gray wisps—stale thoughts, drained emotions, even other people's energies that cling like burrs. See these wisps dissolve harmlessly into the larger atmosphere, transformed into neutral energy by the radiance you have summoned.

After several cycles, notice the edge of your aura. At first it may feel ragged or inconsistent. As you continue, the boundary evens out. Some describe a sensation like the gentle push of air when two magnets repel each other; others feel warmth or tingling. Pay attention to any areas where the Healing Wave seems to skip or dims prematurely. These are likely micro-fissures, the tiny tears we discussed earlier in the book. You can linger there for an extra breath or two, perhaps visualizing the light as needle and thread, stitching the gap before continuing.

Practice the Healing Wave for ten to fifteen minutes. When you finish, let the imagery dissolve slowly. Open your eyes, taking note of colors, shapes, and sounds in the room. Ground yourself by rubbing your palms together and pressing them against your heart or solar plexus. This seals the repair work, the way a doctor applies a protective dressing after suturing.

Chakra-Aligned Breathing: Feeding the Rainbow

The Complete Guide to Aura Healing

You already know that each chakra radiates a corresponding hue into the auric layers. When a chakra is sluggish, the color in that region of the aura appears dull or thin. Chakra-aligned breathing directly feeds prana to these energy centers, brightening the associated fields.

Start with breath awareness. On your next inhale, draw cool, luminous red into the base of the spine, the root chakra. Imagine the red swirling like liquid ember. As you exhale, allow that red to expand outward into the area around your hips and lower torso, saturating the aura there.

Move up to the sacral chakra, breathing in a vibrant orange that pools below the navel, then radiates on the exhale. Continue through the spectrum: yellow in the solar plexus, green in the heart, sky blue in the throat, indigo in the third eye, and violet or white at the crown. Spend two to three cycles on each chakra before ascending to the next. When you reach the crown, picture all seven colors spiraling together like a sunlit prism. On the final exhale, let this multicolored spiral expand far beyond the physical body until you are enclosed in a swirling rainbow sphere.

I once guided a client named Akiko through this practice after she came to me complaining of persistent throat infections and chronic self-doubt. After three weeks of daily chakra-aligned breathing, not only did her physical symptoms subside, but she reported confidently presenting her artwork at a local gallery opening—something she had postponed for years. The throat chakra's bloom illuminated her aura, and that amplified presence rippled into her outer life.

The Central Channel Meditation: Repairing the Core

Every aura has a central axis, often called the sushumna in yogic literature or antahkarana in esoteric traditions. Visualize it as a slender vertical highway along which your chakras align. When this channel is clear, the aura maintains structural integrity; when blocked, the field warps. The Central Channel Meditation clears and reinforces this highway.

Settle into breath awareness. With a gentle inhale, draw a thread of silver-white light up from the earth's crystalline heart through your root chakra into the center of your chest. With the next inhale, draw golden light from the sun through your crown to meet the silver thread in the heart. Feel the two lights weave together, forming a luminous rope that within a few breaths extends from earth to sky straight through your body. As you breathe, sense microscopic filaments extending from this rope, binding any loose or frayed auric fibers back toward center, much like a maypole gathering ribbons.

Within a week of consistent practice most people report a distinct vertical stability, as if an inner compass realigns itself. One student, Jonah, described feeling "taller on the inside," and his friends noticed he carried himself with unusual poise. His aura photographs taken before and after a month of Central Channel Meditation revealed a striking straightening of colors that had previously sagged to one side.

The Torus Field Technique: Advanced Expansion

If the aura appears egg-shaped on casual inspection, sensitive perception often discovers a more dynamic torus field — a donut-shaped flow rising through the spine, arcing outward above the head, descending around the body, and curving back up through the feet. Engaging the torus can dramatically enhance energetic circulation.

Begin in a seated posture. Inhale, feeling energy rise up the spine like water in a fountain. At the crown, imagine the stream arching forward, cascading outward in a slow-motion waterfall. Exhale as the energy descends in a gentle curve in front of the body down to the feet, then imagine it sweeping under the soles and re-entering up through the back body to rejoin the spine. Continue breathing, visualizing a perpetual loop. With practice the sensation grows visceral; several practitioners liken it to sitting within a softly rotating magnetic field.

During my sabbatical in Costa Rica I taught this method to a circle of surfers who wanted quicker recovery from muscle fatigue. Within a fortnight they reported not only less soreness but an uncanny intuition of timing waves. When the torus spun evenly, their peripheral awareness sharpened, allowing them to read the ocean's subtle cues—an outer analog to detecting shifts in the auric sea.

Color-Infused Breath for Specific Repairs

Sometimes an aura sports localized bruises: a specific limb encased in a muddy hue after injury, or a dull patch hovering near a grieving heart. Color-infused breath allows you to target these zones much like a skilled restorer matches paint to a damaged fresco.

Begin with the Healing Wave to establish a receptive field. Then identify the damaged area. Suppose a friend's cutting remark still stings in your upper chest, leaving a gray smudge. Inhale emerald green light—symbolic of unconditional love—directly into that patch. Hold softly, picturing the green swirling, soaking, scrubbing. Exhale, releasing soot-colored debris. Repeat until the green saturates evenly and the emotional ache subsides.

I once used this approach to heal a persistent ache in my left shoulder that followed an intense period of caregiving for a terminally ill relative. Medically, nothing was wrong; emotionally, I carried the weight of unexpressed grief. After a week of directing indigo-flecked blue (communication and release) into the shoulder during breath meditation, I woke one morning to find both the ache and a long-standing sense of burden had melted.

Heart Coherence Meditation: The Compassion Engine

If the aura had a command center, it would arguably be the heart field. Heart-math studies reveal that the electromagnetic field produced by the heart is sixty times more powerful than that of the brain. Synchronizing breath and emotion at the heart — a state called coherence — produces a harmonic signature that radiates throughout the aura like a tuning fork.

Close the eyes and rest a hand over the sternum. Begin slow, even breaths: five seconds in, five seconds out. As you breathe, recall a memory or imagine a scenario that evokes genuine appreciation. The moment the feeling arises, amplify it on the inhale as though drawing warm rose light into the chest. On the exhale, let that rose light pulse outward through every auric layer, soft but insistent, like ripples in a pond. After a few minutes you may experience a palpable buoyancy around your skin, as though cushions of air support you.

When my niece Amelia faced bullying in middle school, we practiced heart coherence together each evening via video call. She imagined hugging her golden retriever while breathing. Within days her mother noted Amelia carried an unmistakable glow that discouraged further teasing; her aura broadcast calm confidence classmates seemed reluctant to rattle.

Sounded Breath: Humming, Toning, and the Aura

Sound is rhythm made visible in the aura. You observed in Chapter 14 how tuning forks and singing bowls organize chaotic fields; when you produce sound with your own vocal cords, the effect is immediate and personal. Combine that vibration with intentional breathing and you create what I call Sounded Breath.

Take a comfortable inhale. On the exhale, allow a soft hum to escape, lips closed, resonating primarily in the chest. Feel the vibration spread through tissues into the auric layers. Next cycle, shape your mouth into an open "ah" and let the vibration rise into the head, then spill outward. Alternate between hums and open tones for five minutes. Each sound wave acts like sonar, mapping and smoothing hidden rough patches in the aura.

I have observed that people who feel socially invisible often experience an almost translucent aura. Sounded Breath thickens the field, making them more perceptible to others. A shy college student named Priya practiced daily humming and reported that when she entered seminar rooms classmates simply "noticed me more," without her needing to speak louder. Her aura had quite literally become more audible.

Mantra-Infused Breathing: Programming the Light

A mantra is a phrase laden with specific vibratory meaning. Repeating it on the breath inscribes that meaning into the auric matrix. Choose a mantra that resonates with your healing intent. If Sanskrit calls to you, "So Hum" (I am That) is elegant; if plain English feels honest, try "I am whole." Whisper the mantra on each exhale, receiving silent stillness on each inhale. The aura, sensitive as photographic film, records every impression. Within a fortnight the mantra carves grooves of coherence; random static has less room to settle.

During my own convalescence from pneumonia, I used the seed sound "Ram"—associated with the solar plexus—to rebuild depleted vitality. Coupled with measured breathing, the mantra felt like a smith's hammer forging fresh armor around a previously threadbare area of my aura. Medical recovery accelerated, but just as valuable was the renewed courage that bloomed once the solar plexus fired bright again.

Navigating Obstacles: The Restless Mind and Body

Not every session will feel celestial. Sometimes knees ache, the neighbor's dog barks, or your brain insists on cataloging grocery lists. That does not mean failure; it means you are alive. Accept small disruptions as part of the practice. Each return to the breath is a micro-victory, reinforcing neural circuits of presence. If physical pain is the issue, adjust your posture or use props—not as indulgence, but as intelligent strategy to keep your aura relaxed. If emotion swells unexpectedly, treat it as surfacing debris the Healing Wave has dislodged. Breathe through the sensation, neither suppressing nor amplifying. Most emotions crest and fall within ninety seconds if unresisted.

Remember that auric healing is non-linear. One day you may feel enormous expansion; the next, apparent constriction. Picture a snake shedding skin: before the new layer glistens, the old must crack, which can feel tight. Trust the process and continue breathing light into any tightness.

Case Story: Maria's Postpartum Renewal

Maria, a thirty-three-year-old teacher, came to see me seven months after giving birth. She described crippling fatigue and an aura she sensed as "patched with duct tape." During intake I noticed a significant dimming around her sacral and heart regions, common after the intense physiological and emotional demands of childbirth.

We began with foundational breath awareness to rebuild baseline vitality. By week two, she incorporated the Healing Wave, focusing extra breaths on her lower abdomen. Week four introduced heart coherence to address emotional depletion, and by week six, Sounded Breath using the mantra "Ma" on exhale to honor maternal identity.

At week eight Maria surprised herself by jogging for the first time since pregnancy, feeling lighter than she had in years. Color-reading photography before and after the program revealed a pronounced increase in orange and green hues, signifying rejuvenated creative and heart energies. Maria's testimonial still gladdens me: "My aura no longer feels like duct-taped glass; it feels like a living, breathing sunrise." Her story illustrates how layered breath-based practices can restore structural integrity and luminosity even after significant life events.

Weaving Practice into Everyday Life

A question invariably arises: "How do I keep this up when life gets hectic?" My answer is: shrink the practice without diluting its essence. The breath lives in every moment; you need not reserve healing solely for the cushion.

While waiting at a traffic light, you can perform two cycles of Chakra-Aligned Breathing, perhaps focusing on the solar plexus if stress looms. Standing in line for coffee becomes an opportunity for Heart Coherence, recalling a loved one and sending rose light into the aura. Before sleep, lie on your back and allow the Torus Field Technique to cradle you, the gentle loop lulling the nervous system into deeper rest. These miniature sessions stitch continuity through your day, ensuring the aura remains supple rather than swinging between extremes of expansion and neglect.

Safety and Ethical Considerations

Some advanced breathwork styles promoted elsewhere—such as prolonged hyperventilation—can provoke dizziness or emotional flooding. If you are pregnant, have cardiovascular issues, or a history of panic attacks, consult a qualified healthcare professional and employ gentler variations. Remember also that an aura, once brightened, becomes more sensitive to subtle influences, much like newly exfoliated skin. Avoid immediately plunging into chaotic environments. Give your field time to stabilize; you may even layer in the protective shields described in the previous chapter until you sense equilibrium.

Finally, respect others' energy boundaries. A powerful aura can unconsciously dominate space. Breathe radiance for collective uplift, not for egoic display. Genuine strength arrives quiet and inclusive.

Conclusion: Breathing Life into Connection

By now you can feel how meditation and breathwork sustain the inner climate from which all aura repair arises. You have practiced drawing light into torn places, spinning color through dull patches, and harmonizing your heart's rhythm with the rhythm of breath. Each technique is a brushstroke; together they paint a living masterpiece that is your renewed energy field.

In the next chapter we will explore how this strengthened, coherent aura interacts with the people around you. Breathing is inherently relational; every exhale becomes somebody else's inhale, every thought-formed vibration reverberates across invisible bridges. As you step from solitary practice into the rich tapestry of relationships, your revitalized aura will both influence and be influenced. Let us now examine that exchange with the same attentiveness we have given to your breath, and learn to dance consciously with the countless other fields that surround you.

Chapter 17 - Energy Exchange: Relationships and Your Aura

A Quiet Current Between Us

When you finished the breathwork exercise at the close of the previous chapter, you may have felt a subtle hum in and around your body—an echo of your own life force, steady and certain. Now imagine that hum settling into a room filled with other people, each carrying a vibration uniquely their own. Without words, you begin to sense who feels calming, who feels electrifying, and who seems to muddy the air around them. That wordless sensing is the focus of this chapter: the continuous flow of energy between you and everyone you meet. Just as you exchange oxygen and carbon dioxide with a houseplant, you also exchange energetic information—sometimes nourishing, sometimes depleting, always influential.

I want to guide you through this invisible dialogue, because understanding it will empower you to protect your well-being, nurture deeper intimacy, and, when necessary, walk away with clarity rather than guilt. Over years of private practice I have seen people transform debilitating relationship patterns simply by tending to the space two feet beyond their skin. By the time you finish this chapter, you will know how to recognize energetic exchanges in real time, how to repair damage they may cause, and how to cultivate relationships that lift everyone involved.

The Invisible Conversation—How Auras Communicate

Science has known for decades that electromagnetic fields extend from the heart, the brain, and even the DNA inside each cell. Spiritual traditions have long described luminous bodies radiating farther than the eye can see. In daily life you experience the overlap of those fields every time you lean in during a heartfelt talk or recoil from someone who "rubs you the wrong way." Your aura behaves like a sensitive membrane that both emits and receives signals.

I often picture two soap bubbles drifting toward one another. As soon as they touch, their glossy surfaces stretch, merge, and sometimes pop. The same happens to your energy field. A casual brush with a stranger on the subway is a brief, almost imperceptible contact—a whisper of information. A hug from a long-time friend is a prolonged merging that can either fortify or drain. And an intimate relationship? That is more like two bubbles partially fusing, creating a new surface you share.

You don't have to do anything deliberate to initiate these exchanges. Energy fields seek equilibrium, so the moment you enter someone's space, their field samples yours and vice versa. Yet you do have a choice about how long you stay in contact, how porous you allow your field to become, and how fully you invite another's energy inside. Recognizing this choice is the first step to mastering relational aura health.

Science and Mysticism of Interpersonal Energy

When the HeartMath Institute measured heart-generated magnetic fields, researchers found those fields could be detected several feet away with sensitive equipment. They also demonstrated that one person's coherent heart rhythm—achieved through gratitude or loving thoughts—could induce coherence in another's heart pattern, even without touch or conversation. Mystics describe the same influence in more poetic terms, calling it entrainment or resonance.

In my early twenties I attended weekly meditation sittings led by a teacher whose presence felt remarkably still. Before she spoke a single word, I noticed my own chaotic thoughts settling, as though my mind were a violin adjusting to her tuning fork. HeartMath supplied the charts; my lived experience supplied the certainty. That teacher's aura entrained mine every Wednesday night, and for several days afterward my interactions with coworkers were kinder, my decisions clearer. Energy exchange isn't limited to the esoteric—it shows up in boardrooms, bedrooms, and grocery store lines.

Recognizing Energetic Signatures—Why Some People Feel Familiar

Have you ever met someone for the first time and felt as though you already knew them? That sense of familiarity isn't always past-life mystique; often it's the simple fact that their energetic pattern echoes one you have encountered before. Children raised by anxious parents, for example, develop a vibratory "ear" for jittery fields. Later, when they meet a stranger whose aura buzzes at that same tempo, they subconsciously recognize the frequency. Familiarity feels like safety—even if the original experience was not safe at all.

One client, Mara, continually fell into friendships with people who devalued her time. She found herself answering late-night crisis calls, rewriting résumés, even babysitting pets on zero notice. When we explored her childhood, she realized that her mother's aura was perpetually frazzled, demanding unseen labor from everyone nearby. Mara had come to equate that frenetic buzz with belonging. The day she sensed the same buzz in a new acquaintance's field, she smiled politely, excused herself, and later remarked, "For the first time, I knew the difference between recognition and resonance."

Learning to identify these signatures allows you to pause before entangling. Does this person's energy raise your baseline or disturb it? Instead of asking whether you like someone, invite your body to tell you how their field affects your own. Your aura, not your intellect, is often the better judge.

Cord Connections—Healthy Bonds and Draining Tethers

Every meaningful relationship creates energetic cords—strands of condensed information that carry emotion, memory, and intent. Imagine them as fiber-optic cables flashing signals back and forth. When cords are balanced, both people feel supported. Parents and infants share thick, luminous cords that gradually thin as the child matures, allowing autonomy. Lovers establish cords at the heart, solar plexus, and sometimes sacral chakras, blending desire, power, and compassion. Close friends often cord at the throat, exchanging unfiltered truths.

Cords become destructive when they clamp rather than connect. If one person fears abandonment, their cords might hook into the other's field with a desperate grip, siphoning energy to soothe an inner void. The recipient may feel inexplicably tired or irritable after short conversations. I once counseled two sisters: the elder, Beth, was rebuilding her life after divorce; the younger, Liv, overflowed with caretaking instinct. Liv's cords latched onto Beth's heart center so tightly that Beth reported chest heaviness each time her phone buzzed with Liv's name. By teaching Liv to anchor her sense of purpose within her own body, and Beth to visualize a gentle unhooking without rejecting her sister's love, we restored mutual nourishment.

You needn't sever every challenging cord—some simply require adjustment, like loosening a too-tight guitar string until it sings again.

Empathy, Sympathy, and the Hazards of Over-Merging

Empathy is the ability to feel what another feels; sympathy is the ability to care about what another feels. Both become hazardous when you lose track of which feelings belong to whom. As an empathic psychotherapist, I used to finish sessions with a headache behind my eyes. I attributed it to screen fatigue from taking notes, yet on vacation the headaches vanished. I eventually realized that my third-eye chakra was oversaturated from absorbing client sorrow I had not processed in my own field.

Energetic over-merging often masquerades as kindness. You might believe you are lightening a friend's burden by carrying her anger about a breakup, when in fact you're denying her the cathartic release she needs to process that anger herself. Over-merging also cripples discernment. If you adopt a colleague's anxiety, you may misinterpret it as a sign you should flee a project, when the truth is it isn't your fear at all.

The remedy is compassionate differentiation: standing close enough to witness, but rooted deeply enough in your own aura that you recognize the border. Picture your field as a shoreline. You can let someone dip their toes in the tide without inviting them to build a house on the sand.

Romantic Relationships and Aura Co-Regulation

Few arenas highlight energetic exchange more vividly than romance. From the euphoria of new love to the aching tension of unspoken resentment, couples continuously co-regulate each other's fields. Early infatuation often produces a rosy glow—literally, pinkish tones appear in the auric field as affection heightens. Hormones flood the bloodstream, expanding the heart chakra and thinning the boundary between partners. Everything the other does seems extraordinary because you are reading their field almost as your own.

As novelty fades, individual rhythms reassert themselves. That is when many couples confront differences they assumed did not exist. The challenge is to maintain a healthy overlap—enough fusion to feel bonded, enough differentiation to breathe freely. In my own marriage, I notice that if we discuss finances late at night, my husband's pragmatic earth-toned field grounds me, but it can also dampen my creative gold shimmer. We schedule logistical talks in the morning now, when my gold is naturally subdued and his earthy calm feels stabilizing rather than oppressive.

Sexual intimacy compounds these effects. The root and sacral chakras open wide, releasing potent currents that linger for up to forty-eight hours. During that window partners are unusually susceptible to each other's moods. A careless remark can penetrate more deeply; a loving affirmation can reverberate with amplified healing. Knowing this, you can turn lovemaking into an intentional energy medicine session: set an intention together, visualize colors blending, and rest in stillness afterward, allowing your fields to integrate the experience.

Family Systems—Inherited Patterns in the Field

Families do not merely pass down eye color and holiday recipes. They transmit vibrational blueprints, sometimes across centuries. If your grandparents survived war or famine, the survival frequency they cultivated—contracted auras, vigilant solar plexus chakras—may still hum in your cells. You might call yourself cautious or risk-averse without realizing you are echoing a trauma that predates you.

I worked with a client, Devon, whose aura flared crimson whenever someone challenged him, even playfully. Intrigued, he traced the family lineage and discovered that his great-grandfather, a labor organizer, had been beaten for defying factory owners. Devon's field was reliving the need to fight. Through guided visualization, he thanked his ancestors for their protection, then invited the crimson flare to soften into a warm orange of creative problem-solving. Within weeks his colleagues described him as more approachable, and he felt lighter, as though a heavy coat had slipped from his shoulders.

Family fields can be empowering too. A lineage of musicians may endow descendants with spinning turquoise spirals at the throat, making self-expression effortless. By acknowledging inherited patterns, you choose which to cultivate and which to release.

Friendship and Community—Circles of Mutual Amplification

When several coherent auras gather with a shared purpose, the collective field magnifies exponentially. Religious services, protest marches, book clubs—each creates a group aura. You have probably left a concert still singing, heart pounding with communal resonance. That afterglow is evidence of your field vibrating at the memory of collective joy.

A personal example: I host quarterly women's circles for moon rituals. We begin separately, tuning into individual intentions. By the time we reach the candle-lighting, I can feel our auras weaving into a luminous quilt overhead. Two hours later participants walk out nourished yet light, as though they have emptied burdens into the fire and pocketed sparks of inspiration in return. The gift of community is amplification without depletion.

To sustain such circles, each member must arrive willing to contribute authentic energy rather than siphon from the group. You will learn to recognize difference in sensation: amplification feels expansive and buoyant; siphoning feels heavy and dull. Trust your body's report card.

Professional Interactions—Energetic Boundaries at Work

Workplaces are petri dishes of clashing and complementary auras. Open-plan offices encourage fields to intermingle all day, which can inadvertently replicate the family table—complete with sibling rivalries and parental authority shadows. Many clients say they feel "fried" after meetings where opinions ricochet. What they are sensing is excess mental energy—sharp citrine tones of the third-eye chakra without grounding red from the root.

During my corporate training years, I traveled weekly and often entered conference rooms buzzing with anticipation. I learned a small trick: as I set my laptop on the table, I silently extended a sheet of cobalt blue light four inches beyond my skin. That buffer absorbed stray stimuli so I could lead with clarity. Colleagues described me as calm under pressure, unaware that the calm was a boundary made visible only to me.

You, too, can practice boundary hygiene at work by starting the day anchored in your own field, checking in during breaks, and cleansing before you leave the parking lot. In doing so, you will commune from choice rather than compulsion.

Conflict, Trauma, and Repair—Healing Aura Wounds in Relationship

Conflict is inevitable wherever two sovereign beings intersect. Yet conflict need not scar your aura irreparably. What injures the field is not the disagreement itself but the unresolved emotional charge trapped afterward. Picture two dancers who misstep and collide. If they stop, breathe, and adjust, harmony resumes. If they keep dancing while nursing bruised egos, the tension multiplies and eventually tears fabric.

When my friend Jonah ended a business partnership abruptly, the partner sent scathing emails. Jonah could have mirrored the anger, but instead he visualized a violet flame dissolving cords of resentment each morning. He still responded to emails—in concise, respectful language—but the flames burned away the emotional debris. Months later, the ex-partner apologized for lashing out, and both moved on unburdened.

Repair requires acknowledgment, not perfection. Say the hard truth, own your energy, invite the other to own theirs, and then consciously restore the field. Sometimes that involves conversation; other times silent prayer suffices. The key is intention followed by embodiment.

Conscious Energy Exchange—Intentional Practices for Healthy Boundaries

Imagine standing with a friend, eyes closed, palms a few inches apart. You feel warmth pulsing between you—proof that energy follows awareness. Now imagine amplifying that warmth with deliberate breath, letting it circulate like water in a fountain that nourishes both without draining either. Intentional exchange is that simple.

Start by grounding yourself: feet on the floor, spine long, breath slow. Invite your aura to fill every corner of your body and extend naturally outward. Only then do you open to the other person's presence. When the visit concludes, thank them silently, recall your breath, and gather your field back to its resting size. Over time this ritual becomes second nature, a courtesy as automatic as shaking hands.

During more complex encounters—family holidays, staff evaluations—you can pre-set your field to a current of compassion or curiosity, much like tuning a radio station before the show begins. Others will sense the clarity and often match it unconsciously.

Self-Inquiry: Am I Giving or Receiving?—Balance of Flow

Energy exchange is healthiest when flow is bidirectional and proportionate. Like tides, sometimes you will give more, sometimes receive more, but over the season balance should return. To evaluate, pause regularly and ask: Do I feel fuller or emptier after this interaction? If emptier, did I consciously choose to pour into the other, and do I have a plan to refill? If fuller, am I grateful without guilt?

During my mother's illness, I chose to give more energy than I received, fully aware that caregiving is a temporary season. I scheduled weekly acupuncture and forest walks to replenish. Because the imbalance was conscious and my self-care intentional, resentment never took root. Unconscious imbalance breeds fatigue and, eventually, bitterness.

Your aura keeps score even when you don't. Learn its language, and it will guide you toward equitable flow.

Case Study: The Therapist and Empathic Burnout

Elena, a social worker, arrived in my office defeated. Ten years into her career, she loved her clients yet dreaded Mondays. Her aura, once turquoise and bright, had dulled to a chalky gray. She confessed that she replayed each client story at home, often dreaming their nightmares as though they were her own.

We began with daily closure rituals: after the final session she imagined placing each client in a bubble of golden light, sealing it, and handing it to their higher self. Then she brushed her arms from shoulders to fingertips, shaking off residue like water. Within a month her turquoise returned. She started painting again, a hobby she had abandoned. The dreams ceased. Elena's field was not the problem; her unsupervised permeability was. By reclaiming the membrane, she rediscovered joy in service without sacrificial cost.

Case Study: A Couple Rebalancing Their Fields

Marcus and Priya appeared for joint aura counseling after three years of escalating arguments. Marcus felt smothered; Priya felt abandoned. Energy scans revealed Marcus's heart chakra retracting whenever Priya approached, while Priya's solar plexus flared, attempting to pull him back. We designed a simple practice: before discussing sensitive topics, they sat back-to-back, eyes closed, breathing in sync for five minutes. The lack of eye contact relieved pressure; the shared rhythm re-established subtle connection.

By week three, Marcus's heart field warmed to a soft emerald even face-to-face, and Priya's solar plexus quieted. Their conversations shifted from accusations to invitations. Physical space coupled with energetic attunement created safety to re-engage. The practice became a nightly ritual long after therapy ended, a living reminder that balanced fields nourish love better than words alone.

Clearing After Connection—Daily Rituals

Brains favor repetition, and so do energy fields. The simplest daily habits accumulate profound impact. At dusk I step outside, inhale sky, and exhale any energy not mine. On busier days I add a gentle sweep of my aura with a feather fan by the door, thanking each interaction for its lessons. What matters most is consistency, not complexity. Choose a time—shower, commute, twilight, or pillow—and declare it your clearing point. Your field will quickly associate that moment with relief, relaxing like feet slipping into familiar slippers.

When Separation Heals—Ending Toxic Ties

Despite your best efforts, some relationships erode well-being. In such cases, physical and energetic separation is medicine, not failure. Ending a toxic friendship, dissolving a business partnership, or filing for divorce all require courageous boundary setting followed by cord clearing.

After my own difficult breakup in my late teens, I discovered a ritual that remains my compass: I visualized a crystal dagger cutting cords at the solar plexus, then placed rose petals on both ends, symbolizing gratitude for what was learned. Each morning for a month I repeated the cut and the blessing. By day thirty my stomach unclenched, and I could recall the relationship with appreciation rather than pain. Separation healed what continual contact could not.

Seamless Currents—Transitioning to Your Environment

As you tune your relationships, remember that energy exchange is never limited to people. The spaces you inhabit—your home, office, street, and city—also pulse with fields that can nourish or deplete. In the next chapter we will explore how walls, furniture, technology, and even the land beneath your feet interact with your aura. The skills you have honed here will serve you there, for boundaries with places are crafted in the same language of awareness, intention, and flow.

Close your eyes now and sense the echo of every human interaction you experienced today. Feel where those echoes rest in your field, then invite any discordant notes to release on the next exhale. Your aura hums, clear and centered, ready to dance with the environments that await.

The Complete Guide to Aura Healing

Chapter 18 - Environmental Influences on Your Energy Field

Bridging Relationships and Place

In the last chapter, you and I explored how the threads of relationship weave in and out of your aura, sometimes nourishing it, sometimes fraying its edges. It was an intimate discussion about the people who lean close to your field, the cords they attach, and the boundaries you sculpt. Yet relationship does not end with human contact. The moment you step beyond another's embrace, your aura continues its dialogue—this time with everything around you: the walls, the trees, the hum of traffic, the scent of rain-soaked soil, even the unseen electromagnetic pulses that quiver through modern life. Every place has a personality, an energy signature that rises up to meet your own. Understanding that conversation between you and your environment is the next logical step on our journey, and that is exactly where this chapter leads us.

The Energetic Echo of Place

Have you ever walked into a room and felt suddenly elated, even though nothing had changed in your personal life within the previous few minutes? Or perhaps you entered a space—an old basement, a cramped office cube, a hospital corridor—and felt an inexplicable heaviness clamp around your chest. That immediate sensorium of mood shift is your aura registering environmental influence before your rational mind can piece together a story. Your energy field is not merely a self-contained bubble; it is a living membrane that constantly absorbs, filters, responds, and broadcasts. Each location, in turn, carries an imprint left by natural features, by the architecture that frames it, and by the emotional residue of the people who most frequently inhabit it.

There is a memorable afternoon I spent in a centuries-old library in Lisbon. I remember running my fingers along shelves polished by generations of scholars and monks. The scent of weathered leather mingled with the soft hush of turning pages. As I stood beneath vaulted ceilings, I noticed my aura expanding in a subtle but unmistakable way. It felt as though invisible hands were stretching a luminous cloak outward from my shoulders, inviting me to breathe more deeply. I later learned that the library's foundation stones had been quarried from local limestone—a porous rock known in energetic anatomy for its capacity to absorb tension. Add to that the quiet reverence of readers concentrated on knowledge rather than anxiety, and you have a space that bathes anyone who enters in an ambient sense of calm curiosity. The point is not that every limestone building will boost your field, nor that every library will refresh you. Rather, it illustrates how the alchemy of material, intention, and human history co-creates an energy climate to which your aura must acclimate.

Physical Space and Aura Density

Let's begin with something measurable: square footage. You already know the sensation of being crammed into a crowded subway train, unsure where your body ends or another's begins. In such moments, your aura is forced to contract. Its layers press inward so it can conserve resources and prevent emotional overload. On the flip side, when you stand alone at the edge of a desert or on the deck of a sailboat, you may notice the field loosening, blooming outward, taking advantage of uncrowded air.

This reflexive adjustment is similar to how your pupils dilate in darkness or shrink under bright sun. The energetic body modulates its density to match perceived safety.

What matters here is awareness. If you find yourself living or working in chronically cramped quarters, your aura may habituate to a constant low-level contraction. Over weeks or months, that can hamper the natural ebb and flow of vital energy and lead to sluggishness, irritability, or emotional reactivity. Conversely, individuals who spend most of their days in wide-open landscapes may struggle to pull their fields inward when intimacy or focused attention is required. I once mentored a young geologist who spent three consecutive seasons mapping volcanic ridges in Iceland. When she returned to city life, she experienced overwhelming sensory inputs at cafés and grocery stores. It took intentional breathwork and grounding exercises to remind her field how to hold its edges in social proximity. Space, then, does not merely shape comfort; it trains your aura's muscularity.

Natural Landscapes: Forests, Oceans, Mountains

Whenever modern life begins to grate, we feel the instinctive tug toward nature. That instinct is more than poetic nostalgia; it is energy hygiene. Each natural landscape supplies a distinct frequency palette that your aura uses like nutritional supplements. Forests hum in rhythm with chlorophyll-rich growth, releasing negative ions that bind to free radicals in your body. I have often taken groups into old-growth woods for weekend retreats. Participants consistently report that their mental chatter quiets within half an hour, and their personal fields attain a velvety texture, as though the forest canopy is brushing away debris that accumulated from city living.

Oceans, with their vast horizons and rhythmic tide, operate on a different bandwidth. Saltwater is a powerful conductor, and the meeting of water and wind produces aerosols that cleanse the aura's outer layers. People who feel emotionally congested often discover a sense of catharsis after simply sitting near crashing surf. There's an anecdote I cherish about a client who had lost his partner. For months he couldn't shake waves of grief that manifested as stagnant grey patches in his auric field. We spent a week together on a quiet section of the Oregon coast. Each dawn, he walked barefoot at the tideline while I guided gentle breathing. By the fourth day, both of us perceived where once there had been a dull haze there was now a shimmering silver-blue band, a sign that sorrow had transmuted into reflective wisdom.

Mountains offer altitude and solidity. Their frequency is slower, grounded by geological mass, yet paradoxically higher in vibration due to thinner atmosphere. If your aura is riddled with too much nervous fire—common among urban professionals—time at elevation delivers a cooling steadiness. Personal story: during a particularly hectic book tour, I scheduled a single free day in the Alps. Hiking above the tree line, I sensed my root chakra plugging into bedrock in a way that felt almost magnetic, while my crown opened to the endless sky. That symmetrical connection recalibrated my entire field for weeks afterward.

Urban Environments and Technological Fields

Cities are symphonies of intersecting energies: human ambition, traffic noise, neon signage, historical memory, concrete density, and not least, electromagnetic radiation from countless devices. Your aura navigates this complexity like a multilingual translator that never sleeps. Some elements can invigorate; others can drain.

Late at night, neon lights flicker with an insistent pulse that forces the subtle body to maintain partial alertness even when you think you are relaxing. Subway tunnels thrum with low-frequency vibrations that can destabilize the root chakra, leading to a vague sense of unease.

Technology deserves specific attention. While the scientific community continues to debate long-term physiological impacts of electromagnetic fields, energy sensitives frequently report auric agitation around Wi-Fi routers, power lines, and cell towers. I am not advocating a total retreat from modern life—most of this manuscript is being written on a laptop, after all—but you can adopt practices that buffer your field. Interior design choices—such as positioning your bed away from large appliances or using fabric impregnated with metallic threads to reflect EMF—are pragmatic. Even more effective is regular grounding: barefoot contact with soil or grass discharges excess static that the aura absorbs from electronics. Think of it as hitting a reset button on your field after a day of screen time.

The social density of cities also introduces emotional cross-pollination. Thousands of overlapping thoughtforms swirl through streets, offices, and subways, each imprinting subtle information. If you are empathic, you may find yourself suddenly irritated or euphoric for no apparent reason. Often the mood you sense is not your own. Shielding techniques from Chapter 15 remain useful, yet there is additional nuance: learning to attune to the city's rhythms can turn potential overwhelm into creative fuel. Artists often thrive in metropolitan centers because the aura, while challenged, also drinks in the inspiration of diverse minds. The trick lies in regular retreat—punctuating urban complexity with quiet sanctuaries, whether that's a rooftop garden, a riverside walkway, or simply a candlelit corner of your apartment where devices are banned.

The Architecture of Energy: Materials, Shapes, Colors

Architecture is frozen music, Goethe declared, and music is vibration. So is architecture. Every material in your home or workplace vibrates at a particular frequency, which interfaces with your aura. Wood, for instance, contains latent life force; it tends to breathe with humidity, subtly expanding and contracting, and that dynamism converses well with the human field. Plastic, by contrast, is largely inert; it can block airflow and hold static charges that irritate the peripheral layers of the aura. Stone conveys elemental gravity; metals channel conductivity. Glass, transparent yet solid, encourages mental clarity but can sometimes contribute to feelings of vulnerability if overused.

Shape matters too. Sharp corners funnel energy into spear-like projections that can pierce auric layers, especially at eye level. Rounded edges allow current to circulate more gracefully. Domes, arches, and spirals echo natural patterns found in shells and galaxies, inviting resonance rather than resistance. I once visited an eco-village in New Mexico where homes were built as geodesic domes from adobe and recycled glass bottles. Residents described unusually vivid dreams and quicker recovery from illness. When I measured their auras with Kirlian photography, I observed fewer ragged edges than typical urban dwellers, and I attribute part of that harmony to the sheltering effect of curved walls.

Color, of course, is frequency made visible. You already learned in Chapter 13 how colored light can heal specific aura layers. Here we focus on ambient color in paint, textiles, and art. Warm tones like terracotta or soft gold stimulate the lower chakras, nurturing security and creativity. Cool tones such as cobalt or forest green soothe the higher layers, promoting introspection. It is not about coating every wall with a single hue. Rather, consider the purpose of each room: a crimson kitchen can invigorate appetite and conversation, while a pale lavender bedroom invites restful sleep and astral journeying. Remember, your aura behaves like a prism. When it encounters a colored environment, it refracts the new wavelength into its own multidimensional palette. Choose with intention, and your surroundings become a personalized healing canvas.

Electromagnetic and Geopathic Stress

Years ago, I was invited to assess the energy in a holistic clinic that reported an uptick of staff fatigue. At first glance, the place seemed idyllic: pastel walls, Himalayan salt lamps, plants thriving in every window. Yet the moment I stepped near the receptionist's desk, my solar plexus contracted sharply. My dowsing rods swung inward, indicating geopathic stress. Further investigation revealed a subterranean water vein intersecting with an underground grid of mineral deposits, creating a natural vortex that siphoned chi. The reception area, unfortunately, sat directly above. We rearranged furniture, introduced a copper rod to ground the swirling current, and within a fortnight staff reported renewed vigor. What looked like burnout had been an environmental drain.

Geopathic stress zones arise where Earth's natural radiation is distorted by subterranean anomalies: watercourses, fault lines, underground cavities, or dense mineral seams. Such anomalies can produce either excess or deficiency in planetary chi, which your aura then has to compensate for. Symptoms may include chronic fatigue, insomnia, headaches, or disrupted concentration. If you suspect such an influence, simple experiments—moving your bed a meter in either direction—can yield immediate relief. Professional dowsers offer more precise mapping, but trust your body first; it is a sensitive instrument.

Electromagnetic stress, meanwhile, is largely human-made. High-voltage power lines, wireless routers, smart meters, and even your trusty cellphone radiate pulsations that overlap with the frequencies your nervous system uses for signaling. When these artificial currents are strong, the aura's natural oscillation can become chaotic. Some individuals develop electromagnetic hypersensitivity, experiencing skin prickles or cognitive fog near electronic devices. Grounding, shielding fabrics, saltwater baths, and strategically placed crystals like black tourmaline are allies. Another overlooked tactic is rhythmic breathing. Slow, diaphragmatic breaths entrain the heart rate variability, which then stabilizes the electromagnetic field that the heart itself generates. Your personal cardio-electromagnetic pulse is remarkably influential on the aura. When it is coherent, external static loses some of its grip.

Soundscapes and Vibrational Atmospheres

Sound is arguably the most direct environmental agent acting on the aura. You already explored sound healing in Chapter 14, but daily ambient noise exerts continuous micro-adjustments on your field. Think of the difference between a morning awakened by birdsong and a morning jarred by a jackhammer. The former encourages the aura's outer layers to undulate in gentle waves; the latter triggers spiky contractions.

I once lived for three months in a fourth-floor apartment overlooking a busy intersection in Buenos Aires. Every evening at seven, two bus lines screeched curbside, belching diesel fumes and horn blasts. During that period, I noticed frayed rips forming in my emotional body, visible as ragged red streaks when I meditated. No matter how diligently I practiced shielding, the constant acoustic assault gnawed away at my field's elasticity. The lesson: sometimes spiritual technique is not enough; physical relocation or architectural intervention—such as installing double-pane windows—becomes necessary.

Conversely, you can employ favorable vibrations to uplift your space. Wind chimes near a window invite air currents to dance with metal or bamboo, releasing harmonic overtones that cleanse stagnation. A gentle fountain adds negative ions via evaporating water while masking abrasive city sounds. Even the hum of a refrigerator, if soft and steady, can create a baseline for the aura to entrain—or annoy it if the frequency is dissonant. Pay attention. Close your eyes in each room of your home and listen not only with ears but with skin. Does the soundscape feel nourishing, neutral, or depleting? Adjust accordingly.

Light, Color, and Circadian Harmony

You and I live beneath an ancient clock: the sun's daily arc and the moon's silvery rotations. Your biology evolved to sync hormonal release, digestion, repair, and even mood to that light cycle. Artificial illumination, though a blessing after dark, can scramble that dialogue between sky and cell. Blue-rich LED screens at night tell your pineal gland it is still afternoon, suppressing melatonin. Your aura, sensitive to subtler amplitude shifts, tries to recalibrate and ends up jittery. Insomnia sets in, and the next day the field lacks resilience.

The remedy begins with awareness. If you must work late on a laptop, install applications that warm screen tones after sunset. Embrace dim, amber lighting in bedrooms. And let dawn greet you:

stepping outside within an hour of sunrise, even for five minutes, resets circadian hormones. When your body clock is synchronized, your aura's layers align like nested Russian dolls, each supporting the next. The clarity this brings is palpable; colors in the peripheral aura turn more vivid, and boundaries hold firm.

Natural light also carries etheric information beyond visible wavelengths. Full-spectrum sunlight contains ultraviolet and infrared rays that feed plant photosynthesis and, indirectly, human vitality through vitamin D synthesis. Infrared warmth penetrates muscles, easing tension that might otherwise impede energy flow. If you live in northern latitudes with long winters, consider infrared saunas or full-spectrum lamps to mimic sunlight's missing frequencies. I have counseled many clients battling seasonal affective disorder; those who combine light therapy with aura cleansing often rebound faster than those using light alone.

Scent, Temperature, and Air Quality

Your nose links directly to the limbic system, the brain's emotional attic. A single whiff of pine can teleport you to childhood hikes; the smell of hospital antiseptic might summon dread. This neurological shortcut means scent influences aura through mood induction. Essential oils such as lavender, frankincense, or eucalyptus not only smell pleasant but carry subtle electrical charges that interact with your energy body. Diffusing oils can therefore refine the frequency of a room. Remember, though, that synthetic fragrances often contain petrochemicals which coat mucous membranes and blunt energy perception. Choose pure botanical sources whenever possible.

Temperature sets the backdrop. Excessive heat causes the aura to expand and thin; you may feel scattered. Cold environments compress layers tightly against the skin, potentially stifling emotional expression. Ideally, you oscillate between warm and cool states, akin to yogic pranayama that alternates inhalation and exhalation. Cold showers, for example, temporarily contract the field, followed by a rebound expansion once warmth returns. This elasticity exercises the aura's resiliency, much like cardiovascular intervals tone the heart.

Air quality is the medium through which your aura breathes. Negative ions generated near waterfalls or after thunderstorms attach to airborne pollutants, sinking them out of respiration range. By contrast, closed indoor spaces accumulate positive ions from electronics and insulation materials, making air feel stuffy even when oxygen is adequate. If you cannot open windows, invest in plants known for air purification—peace lilies, snake plants, pothos. They photosynthesize by day, absorbing volatile organic compounds, and they contribute a gentle vitality to the room's subtle climate. I keep a pothos vine above my writing desk; on days when drafts turn stale, its leaves flag slightly as if to caution me to step outside, reminding me that my aura's wellness is literally intertwined with another organism's.

The Subtle Conversation of Objects and Clutter

Every object whispers a story into the space it inhabits. Heirloom jewelry carries generational memory, mass-produced items often retain factory stress, and gifts can hold residues of the giver's unspoken intentions. A cluttered room therefore becomes an orchestra of clashing narratives, each item tugging at your attention field until cognitive overload bleeds into energetic fatigue. Clutter also obstructs physical pathways through which chi should circulate, creating dead zones where stagnant qi collects. Your aura responds by tightening around the body to protect itself, limiting reach and expressiveness.

I learned the power of object resonance when I inherited my grandmother's sewing chest. Though I cherished it, whenever I entered the guest room where it sat, a melancholy weight pressed on my heart. Eventually, I opened every drawer and discovered scraps of half-finished projects, faded notes written in her declining handwriting—projects she abandoned when arthritis stole her dexterity. Recognizing the sadness imprinted in those fibers, I performed a simple ritual: blessing the cloth, completing one of her pincushions myself, then donating the rest to a quilting circle. The energy shifted instantly. What had felt like silent sorrow now emanated warmth and continuity. Your possessions are not inert; they are narrative nodes that can either nourish or drain you.

Minimalism can be a tonic, but emptiness without intention can feel sterile. What matters is conscious curation: choose items that align with your current life story and future aspirations, cleanse antiques before welcoming them, release what no longer reflects your vibration. When your surroundings portray an authentic narrative, your aura settles into coherence, no longer maintaining defensive postures against incongruent echoes.

Community Fields: Collective Energy of Groups and Places

Beyond physical objects and natural features lies a more diffused yet potent influence: collective consciousness. Sacred sites, war memorials, hospitals, stadiums, schools, prisons—each accrues layers of emotional charge from the masses who gather there. This collective field can uplift or oppress. Consider the hush inside a cathedral: even if you are not religious, your aura often stretches upward, mimicking the nave's verticality, attuning to centuries of prayer saturating stone. Contrast that with the edgy atmosphere at certain bus stations after midnight, where anxiety, impatience, and occasional aggression condense in palpable fog.

During a research expedition to study pilgrimage routes in Spain, I visited a chapel said to contain relics of Saint James. Pilgrims from around the world approached the altar on their knees, tears streaming, hearts open. The cumulative devotion was so thick that my own field dissolved into shimmering gold; I felt simultaneously personal and universal. Such collective uplift can catalyze healing, yet remember that group fields remain porous. After leaving powerful gatherings—concerts, rallies, meditation retreats—your aura might feel either amplified or hollowed out. Integration time is essential. Ground yourself, perhaps with a solitary walk or a quiet meal, before reentering the everyday world.

Neighborhoods and workplaces likewise generate ambient moods. If you move into an apartment building plagued by chronic tenant disputes, the etheric residue may churn restlessly, impacting sleep. Businesses that prioritize employee wellbeing often emit a brighter, clearer atmosphere, which correlates with staff satisfaction. As you grow sensitive, you will detect these subtleties and use them to choose environments that align with your growth trajectory.

Seasonal and Weather Influences

Planetary tilts and weather fronts choreograph massive shifts in magnetism and ionization, which filter through your aura whether you pay attention or not. Spring's upsurge stimulates the etheric layer into vivid greens and yellows, readying you for new projects. Summer's blaze expands the emotional and mental bodies outward, sometimes beyond safe boundaries, leading to vacation romances or impulsive spending. Autumn signals contraction; energies spiral inward toward reflective hues of copper, maroon, and indigo. Winter wraps the auric field in crystalline stillness, encouraging deep introspection and repair.

Weather systems can exaggerate or counterbalance these seasonal tendencies. A thunderstorm, for instance, scrubs the sky with lightning's electrical discharge, releasing negative ions that sharpen aura edges. Many migraine sufferers feel either dread or relief as barometric pressure drops; their aura's sensitivity to voltage changes in the atmosphere triggers physiological responses. Wind, especially in arid climates, scours auric surfaces and can leave you feeling brittle unless you moisturize from within through hydration and calming breath. Fog blurs visual and energetic boundaries alike, inviting the psychic realm to drift closer to waking consciousness.

There is no "good" or "bad" weather, only appropriate adaptation. By aligning daily routines with meteorological cues, you train your aura to dance with rather than resist nature's steps. If a heatwave looms, schedule restorative yin yoga, cooling foods, and deeper meditations. When winter's darkness arrives, amplify candlelight, fragrant soups, and communal storytelling. Living seasonally makes your aura supple, responsive, and resilient.

Sacred Sites and Power Spots

Throughout history, humans have identified places where the veil between physical and subtle realms seems thinnest: Stonehenge, Machu Picchu, Uluru, Mount Shasta, Chartres Cathedral. Often these sites rest on ley line intersections or unique geological formations that channel planetary kundalini. Visiting such locales can realign your aura with global energy currents—like syncing your watch to Greenwich Mean Time.

During my pilgrimage to Mount Kōya in Japan, I experienced how a site's spiritual charge can catalyze accelerated clearing. The night I slept in a shukubō, a temple lodging, dreams erupted like fireworks: ancestral faces, karmic storylines, unresolved grief. I awoke disoriented but lighter, as though monks chanting sutras nearby had vacuumed dense debris from my field. Sacred sites are not casual tourist spots for the energy-aware; they are potent surgeries, and preparation is crucial. Hydration, respectful intention, and post-visit integration rituals ensure the downloads you receive translate into grounded wisdom rather than energetic whiplash.

You need not travel across oceans. Power spots exist in every region: a centuries-old oak grove, a confluence of rivers, a hilltop where locals gather for solstice sunrise. When you stumble upon such a place, you will know by the tingling at your crown or the sudden hush that descends upon your thoughts. Cultivate relationship with these sites: offer biodegradable gifts, meditate, sing, write poems. The Earth loves participatory exchange, and the more you give, the more your aura learns to hum in concert with hers.

Crafting a Supportive Personal Ecosystem

By now you realize that environmental influence is multifaceted: material, spatial, acoustic, electromagnetic, communal. It might feel overwhelming to monitor every variable. Take heart. The goal is not perfection but conscious evolution. Start with the room in which you spend the most time. Observe how your aura reacts upon waking: do you feel porous, armored, or at ease? Track changes after cleaning, rearranging furniture, or introducing a plant. Over days and weeks, your subtle senses sharpen, guiding you to refine lighting, reduce clutter, or add nature sounds.

Remember that your aura is both mirror and magnet. As you heal internal patterns, external environments often shift organically. I recall coaching a software engineer who dreaded her grey cubicle. Together we practiced visualization of her aura filling with golden light. A month later, her manager relocated her to a sunlit desk near a window simply because department seating rotated. Synchronicity often answers inner alignment with outer modifications.

If environmental change seems unattainable—perhaps you share a dorm with messy roommates—focus on portable tools. A pocket-sized crystal, noise-canceling headphones, a tiny vial of essential oil, or a grounding affirmation whispered before meetings can erect a micro-climate within the macro one. Over time, small practices accumulate into a robust protective field that both influences and transcends surroundings.

Harvesting Environmental Wisdom

We have journeyed through forests and skyscrapers, across seasons and architectural blueprints, into the electron dance of Wi-Fi signals and the hushed sanctity of pilgrimage trails. You have discovered that your aura is an ever-listening organ, sampling each scent, light ray, and footstep for information it can translate into vitality—or distress. Awareness bestows choice. When you read the subtle cues emanating from place, you reclaim authorship over how your energy field engages.

In the next chapter, we will witness how individuals just like you have leveraged this knowledge in real life. Their stories illustrate transformation not as abstract principle but as lived experience—proof that when environment and intention align, healing unfolds in astonishing ways. I invite you to carry the insights of this chapter forward, so that as you encounter each new space, you can ask not only, "What does this place look like?" but, "How does this place speak to my energy?" The answers will guide you home, wherever you stand.

Chapter 19 - Case Studies: Transformational Healing Stories

A Doorway into Lived Experience

In the last chapter you and I surveyed the landscapes that surround us and discovered how rooms, buildings, cities, and even the weather imprint themselves on the delicate fabric of the aura. But concepts truly bloom in the mind when we see them embodied in real people. I often say that a single honest story carries more instructional power than a hundred abstract explanations, because stories engage the heart while confirming the intellect. Over the years I have sat with thousands of clients—sometimes in quiet, incense-scented studios, sometimes in the sterile hush of hospitals—and I have watched energy fields recover from bruises, tears, and threadbare exhaustion. Each journey is unique, yet recognizable patterns shine through like well-loved constellations.

The six stories you are about to read were chosen because together they form a panoramic view of what aura healing can accomplish. They differ in age, culture, circumstance, and presenting problem, but every one of them ended in a profound shift that rippled outward into family systems, careers, and communities. I recount them here exactly as they happened, with identifying details changed to preserve privacy. As you move through these narratives, I invite you to imagine that you are in the room with me, watching colors swirl and condense, feeling frequencies rise, noticing subtle heat or coolness on the skin. Let these stories be mirrors, windows, and guideposts all at once, for they carry the distilled essence of the techniques we have practiced together throughout this book.

From Burnout to Brilliance: Maya's Homecoming to Herself

Maya was the kind of elementary-school teacher every child hopes for: eyes that sparkled with curiosity, a voice that could coax even the shyest student into participation, and an almost magical ability to turn a lesson about fractions into a treasure hunt. When she booked her first session, however, the sparkle was gone. She moved with the careful slowness of someone carrying a cup filled to the brim, afraid that one unexpected jostle would send everything spilling. Her words tumbled out in anxious rushes: relentless headaches, insomnia, and a vague but persistent sense that she was "fading."

When I attuned to her field, the fading took literal form. The auric layers closest to her body retained some density, but the outer mental and spiritual layers were thinned to gauze, and along her left shoulder I saw a latticework of tiny holes. The solar plexus chakra pulsed in jagged starts and stops, alternating between a muddy yellow and a greenish brown—classic markers of chronic self-doubt and emotional depletion. Maya confirmed what her aura revealed: she felt unseen by administrators, over-accessible to students and parents, and guilty whenever she took even a single personal day.

Our plan unfolded over eight sessions. We began every meeting by cleansing with smoke from dried rosemary and lavender—plants that Maya remembered her grandmother burning in the family kitchen on stressful holidays. Re-establishing this sensory link to a childhood memory allowed her parasympathetic nervous system to soften almost instantly. Once the aura was clear of superficial debris, I used lapis lazuli stones placed gently above her collarbones to seal the lattice of holes. Lapis resonates with the throat and third-eye chakras, and although the damage appeared in her shoulder, it originated in her difficulty speaking needs aloud.

Midway through the course of treatment Maya chose to experiment with a newly learned boundary affirmation. One morning before class she closed her eyes, envisioned a shimmering cobalt sphere around her torso, and whispered, "My energy is mine to steward. I share it consciously and replenish it faithfully." The day was predictably chaotic—two students argued; a parent dropped by unannounced—but that evening she realized she felt only normal fatigue rather than bone-deep exhaustion. Slowly, color returned to her face. The solar plexus chakra brightened each week, shedding the stagnant overtones of brown. By session eight her mental layer looked like wavy amber glass, translucent yet resilient.

The turning point, she told me later, was not a single exercise. It was the dawning comprehension that saying "no" was an act of love toward herself and her students because a befogged teacher cannot deliver clarity. Six months after we completed work, I received a postcard. On the front was a photograph of Maya hiking in Peru. On the back she wrote, "I learned to carry only what belongs to me. Everything feels luminous now."

Maya's story demonstrates how minor structural disruptions—in her case, those delicate holes near the shoulder—can create disproportionate fatigue if they coincide with emotional self-neglect. You can cleanse, repair, and protect, but integration happens when behavior and belief shift. The aura enthusiastically mirrors that new internal stance.

The Architect and the Shattered Shield: Julian's Passage through Grief

Julian entered my practice after spending the better part of a year caring for his dying father. He was an architect known for sweeping, light-filled spaces, yet lately he felt unable to summon any inspiration. Immediately I sensed a heavy drag around him, almost as if he were wading through syrup. Visually, his etheric layer clung close, darker than I typically see in healthy individuals. Two vertical fissures knifed down either side of his chest, starting at the heart chakra and extending outward. These splits revealed raw, sparking edges that alternated between crimson and charcoal gray, indicating both acute sorrow and suppressed anger.

We spent the first session in silence, except for the resonant hum of a 528-Hz tuning fork that I activated just above the heart center. After several minutes Julian began to cry, shoulders heaving, the first tears he admitted he had shed since the funeral. Tears are not merely moisture; they are a physical release of biochemical compounds woven through emotion. As saline dripped, the aura itself drank relief.

During subsequent meetings, we used alternating currents of sound and stillness. Crystal singing bowls in the key of F engaged the fractured heart center, while periods of mindful breath anchored the energy as it reknit. I suggested Julian bring personal objects associated with architectural creation: a drafting pencil, a favorite measuring tape, and a piece of limestone salvaged from one of his earliest projects. When these items were placed in a semi-circle at his feet, the aura responded eagerly, threads of silver shooting outward to touch each object. The etheric layer thickened to normal range within four sessions, but the vertical fissures remained, though now their jagged lips glowed rose instead of red.

The true breakthrough arrived when Julian designed a memorial bench for his father's favorite park. He drafted under moonlight, letting intuitive sketches emerge rather than chasing perfection. On the day he showed me the drawings, I witnessed the fissures close like a perfectly aligned zipper. The charcoal undertone vanished. Instead, down the center of his chest beamlike gold light radiated, feeding both his personal field and the room around him.

He later described feeling as though he had retrieved a lost part of himself. From an energetic standpoint, the project served as a soul-level act of service that harmonized grief with purpose. When we last spoke, Julian was preparing a lecture on biophilic design—architecture that integrates plant life—and he laughed easily, energy unfurling around him like unfettered blueprints.

Grief often causes what I call a shattered shield: the aura's outer edges fracture, leaving the heart exposed without the protective buffering that normally prevents emotional overwhelm. Repair is not about patching the shield forcibly; it is about allowing tears, art, and ritual to weave new connective tissue. Julian's field exemplifies the regenerative capacity inherent in every person once the mourning is honored.

Healing the Healer: Dr. Hart's Return to Embodied Compassion

Dr. Evelyn Hart, an emergency-room physician, requested aura work after noticing numbness creeping into her daily interactions. She spoke of moving through code blues and traumatic injuries in a detached haze, worried that compassion fatigue would prematurely end her career. In the scanning phase, I found her crown chakra humming with frenetic velocity—too open, pulling in the pain of every patient—while the root chakra barely registered, appearing as a faint ember. The aura was top-heavy, bright at the upper layers yet quivering in the lower ones, reminiscent of a tree whose branches thrive but whose roots starve.

Rather than default to the usual cleansing sequence, we began with grounding. I invited her to sit with bare feet on a bed of river stones I keep for such purposes. As she breathed deeply, I traced slow figure-eights from her hips down the legs, encouraging energy flow toward the earth. Dr. Hart admitted this felt strangely vulnerable: "I'm always running upstairs, figuratively and literally. Standing still feels risky." Her statement pointed to the core imbalance. She needed to metabolize the constant influx of emergency-room energy, but she had no ritualistic means for doing so.

We integrated a twenty-minute post-shift routine. Each night in the hospital parking garage she placed hands over her abdomen, visualized a vermilion glow, and inhaled through the nose while muttering, "I belong to this body." Exhaling through the mouth, she imagined stress sinking beneath asphalt into subsoil where microorganisms could recycle it. She followed with three lunges, a physician's pragmatic nod to stretching.

In session five I introduced black tourmaline placed behind knees and at the sacrum, forging a temporary protective lattice. The change was immediate: the upper-layer brightness softened, descending in measured waves until the aura appeared evenly distributed. I watched color drain from an over-stimulated indigo at the brow into a richer burgundy along her lower torso. She reported feeling simultaneously heavy and free, two sensations that rarely coexist yet are hallmarks of effective grounding.

Several weeks later Dr. Hart arrived grinning and exhausted, but in a healthy way. She had delivered a premature baby in the ambulance bay, an intense scenario that would previously have left her jittery for days. Instead, she performed her parking-garage ritual and, in her words, "slept like I'd been felled by a tranquilizer dart." Her colleagues noted she was both calmer and more attuned to patients' emotional needs. The ensuing months solidified a new energetic equilibrium. The crown still functioned as a funnel for intuitive diagnostic insight; the difference lay in strong upward-moving columns of ruby red that surged from her feet. The tree now possessed roots as magnificent as its canopy.

Compassion fatigue is a distortion of noble impulse. Repair requires inviting the healer to become the healed, a reversal that re-teaches the aura to circulate sustenance inward before broadcasting outward. Dr. Hart's recovery reminds us that grounding is not a mundane preliminary step. It is a sacred act of survival for those who stand at the juncture of life and death each day.

From Corporate Cage to Creative Flow: Naveen's Liberation

Naveen managed a large tech team in Singapore. His life looked enviable: generous salary, panoramic apartment view, and weekends spent wakeboarding. Yet he emailed me confessing a "constant buzzing in the skull" and a suspicion that he was "living someone else's dream." Videoconferencing during the pandemic proved helpful because I could observe his aura on screen, muted but visible against a white wall. A thin steel-gray band wrapped around his midsection like a chastity belt for the soul. This was no mere stagnation; it was a self-forged cage created by decades of prioritizing social expectation over creative hunger.

We delved into his history. As a child he painted elaborate cityscapes. By high school he abandoned art to pursue engineering, convinced that security trumped passion. The aura preserved this exact timeline: the causal layer, which archives karmic patterns and life purposes, pulsed in dusty sapphire clouds streaked by flashes of neon orange each time he discussed painting. The orange color—representative of sacral creativity—strained against the gray band.

Our sessions combined breath-work with color therapy. First Naveen used slow diaphragmatic breathing to create space, then bathed the midsection in imagined waves of orange light. I encouraged him to move beyond visualization into tactile experience by holding a smooth carnelian stone against the navel. Carnelian resonates with creative fire and lends courage to change.

Gradually he started sketching again, initially five minutes before bed, later spending entire Sundays immersed in acrylics. During one particularly moving session, he described the sensation of the gray belt cracking. Indeed, I witnessed fissures along the band, through which orange ribbons unfurled like banners in wind. The color spread upward to soften the heart chakra from rigid emerald to supple leaf green, and downward into the root where it ignited vitality.

A pivotal moment occurred when his employer offered a promotion that doubled his salary but demanded relocation and even longer hours. Naveen arrived to our meeting pale, torn between fear and yearning. As he spoke, I saw the gray band attempt to re-solidify. We paused, asked the aura itself what it needed. He closed his eyes, hand over carnelian, and after a quiet minute said, "I need to paint a mural, not manage another merger." He declined the promotion, opted for a lateral part-time consultancy, and within months unveiled an eight-meter mural across a community center wall.

The unveiling day was radiant in every sense. Naveen stood before his artwork wearing a simple white shirt, but his aura looked like sunrise: oranges, pinks, golds, intertwined in sinuous loops. The gray belt had dissolved entirely, replaced by a translucent protective film that allowed energy to circulate freely. He claimed he had never felt more alive or more useful. The trade-off humbled him financially, but the creative flow attracted new opportunities: workshop facilitation, art therapy collaborations, and, eventually, a solo exhibition.

Naveen's journey is instructive because it demonstrates how repression of life purpose manifests as energetic constriction, and how loving attention plus incremental action can melt even the tightest bind. Creativity is not frivolous. It is a biological imperative encoded in the sacral layer of every aura, waiting to enliven each corner of existence.

A Teenager's Battle with Chronic Pain: Zoe's Unfolding Strength

Zoe arrived accompanied by her mother, shoulders slumped under a hoodie, maroon nail polish chipped. She suffered from fibromyalgia-like symptoms since age fourteen, now seventeen and missing school frequently. Medical tests returned inconclusive. Her mother hoped holistic work might reduce pain. Adolescents present special considerations because their energy fields undergo rapid flux alongside hormonal change.

I asked Zoe what she envisioned when she thought about her pain. She said, "It's like barbed wire under my skin." Those words echoed in her aura. The etheric layer churned with sharp black-red spikes, particularly around knees and wrists. The emotional layer looked washed-out, as though drained by the constant ache. Yet near the third eye, I noticed a vibrant swirl of indigo and silver, suggesting strong intuitive potential.

We approached gently. First, I taught her a color-to-touch technique: she assigned each pain flare a corresponding hue, then imagined cool liquid turquoise seeping into flare spots. Though skeptical, she practiced because it was "less boring than homework." After three weeks, she admitted the method shortened flares from hours to minutes.

Next, we introduced sound therapy using a playlist Zoe curated herself—mostly indie bands with female vocalists. Music selection by the client increases resonance; the aura recognizes authenticity. She lay on a therapy table, earbuds in, and I traced her meridians with quartz wands. During one session, I heard her giggle mid-song; simultaneously, I witnessed barbed wire dissolve into smoky coils rising above her body before evaporating. Laughter is the body's spontaneous vibration raising agent, outpacing even chanting in some studies.

Transformation accelerated when Zoe began creating digital art on a tablet, depicting what she called "pain monsters" morphing into mythical creatures. This externalization reframed her narrative: pain became an adversary she could befriend or banish through choice. From an energetic view, her sacral chakra brightened, spraying luminescent orange dotted with violet streaks down into the legs. The spikes shrank until only faint shadows remained.

Six months later Zoe joined her school's hiking club. The girl who once struggled to climb stairs summited a local hill at sunrise. She sent me a photo—arms raised, hoodie flapping like wings. The aura in that picture was beyond vibrant; it rippled outward in concentric pink circles, hallmark of self-love. Her pain did not vanish completely, but episodes lessened in frequency and intensity, and when they arose, she wielded tools to meet them with agency.

Chronic pain often correlates with unexpressed or misunderstood energy surges in intuitive teens. Teaching them creative transmutation rather than suppression can convert torment into artistry and empowerment. Zoe's field proves that even wires of agony can be melted into ribbons of possibility.

Elder Wisdom and Final Gifts: Samuel's Peaceful Dimming

Not every aura story ends with vigor and new projects. Some culminate in a gentle fading because the soul prepares to depart. I include Samuel's journey because healing does not always equate to prolonging life; sometimes it means orchestrating a graceful exit.

Samuel, eighty-four, was a retired jazz musician living with terminal congestive heart failure. His daughter requested sessions to ease anxiety and breathlessness. Upon first meeting, Samuel greeted me with a raspy joke and a mischievous grin. Yet his aura whispered fatigue. The mental and spiritual layers were translucent pearl, already stretching outward like sails catching an unseen breeze. The heart chakra pulsed softly, edged in lavender—color of surrender.

We chose minimal intervention. Each session began with me playing recordings of his own performances. Saxophone notes filled the small bedroom, and with them came swells of amber light cascading from his shoulder girdle into the etheric layer. At times he lifted trembling fingers, air-playing phrases. Energy rippled to fingertips, then drifted out like smoke, integrating with the room.

During our fourth visit, Samuel expressed fear of "leaving the family tangled in my mess." Unsettled financial papers weighed on him. I guided a heart-to-root visual: he pictured a column of emerald green descending to the earth, carrying worries to a subterranean vault guarded by ancestors. As he imagined this, his breath deepened, and the aura shifted to a steady rose-gold glow. He drafted a simple handwritten will that evening, witnessed by neighbors.

A week before passing, he asked whether it was wrong to feel ready. I told him that wanting peace is natural. He closed his eyes and sighed, a sound both weary and relieved. From that moment, the aura gradually shrank in diameter, not through collapse but through elegant contraction, like a curtain lowering at concert's end. The night he died, his daughter, Elena, reported waking to faint sax notes though no device played. She entered Samuel's room to find him smiling, head tilted as if hearing applause. The aura was no longer visible, yet the room felt warm, imbued with the lingering timbre of gratitude.

Healing in this context meant aligning bodily, emotional, and spiritual layers so they could disengage smoothly. The absence of struggle is itself evidence of a well-tended energy field. Samuel's story reminds us that the ultimate purpose of aura work is harmony, whether that harmony fuels a new beginning or orchestrates a dignified conclusion.

Interlacing Threads: What the Stories Reveal

Although every narrative unfolded with its own texture, themes weave them into a collective tapestry. First, authentic expression—whether through teaching, architecture, medicine, painting, digital art, or music—acts as a primary nutrient for the aura. When expression is stifled, constriction appears; when expression flourishes, colors brighten and structures heal. Second, the body's sensory memory serves as a shortcut to resilience. Maya's grandmother's herbs, Julian's drafting tools, Dr. Hart's river stones, Naveen's carnelian, Zoe's playlist, and Samuel's sax notes each anchored the healing in lived experience rather than abstract technique.

Third, incremental practice surpasses sporadic intensity. None of these individuals experienced overnight transformation. Repetition taught the aura to trust safety cues and gradually adopt a new baseline. Finally, healing is holistic. Tears, laughter, courageous decisions, logistical paperwork, and restful death all belong in the spectrum we call aura repair. To witness an energy field is to witness life itself in its raw, evolving continuum.

A Personal Reflection

Writing these accounts fills me with a reverent awe that has not diminished over decades. I often feel like a cartographer chronicling journeys across invisible lands. Yet I also remember that I, too, remain a traveler. Each client acts as both mirror and teacher, revealing where my own aura gleams and where it yearns for tending. Whenever you practice the techniques we explored in earlier chapters, you join this lineage of mutual revelation. You become, simultaneously, healer and healed, observer and participant in a cosmic dance whose choreography extends beyond individual lifetimes.

Preparing for Your Own Practice

The next chapter will gather everything we have studied—science, symbolism, cleansing methods, emotional integration, and the lived wisdom of these stories—and shape it into a personalized path you can sustain day after day. Maya, Julian, Dr. Hart, Naveen, Zoe, and Samuel proved that transformation arises when knowledge meets consistent, heartfelt action. Now it is your turn. Together, we will design an aura healing practice tailored to your rhythms, goals, and sacred quirks, ensuring that your energy field not only recovers from damage but thrives in radiant authenticity.

Chapter 20 - Developing Your Personal Aura Healing Practice

The Threshold of Integration

You have traveled a considerable distance with me, moving from foundational concepts to advanced techniques, observing auras, cleansing them, repairing them, protecting them, and even harmonizing them through color, sound, and breath. By now, you have tried at least a handful of the exercises, noticed energetic shifts in your body, and perhaps felt that subtle hum of aliveness around your skin. Yet a question inevitably arises at this stage of the journey: "How do I weave all of this into a way of life?" A practice is more than a collection of techniques. It is a rhythm that carries you through changing seasons, unexpected challenges, and long stretches of ordinary time. This chapter will guide you in shaping that rhythm, so your energy field not only stays intact but steadily evolves in clarity, resilience, and radiance.

Looking Back to Move Forward

Before you design anything new, pause long enough to appreciate where you began. I remember my own turning point vividly. I was standing in a fluorescent-lit grocery aisle examining a box of herbal tea. I had been reading about auras for months but had never tried to sense one. Without thinking, I softened my eyes the way a teacher had described and glanced at the woman beside me. A faint shimmer outlined her shoulders, pale blue like dawn light. My heart thumped. I almost dropped the tea. The experience was so subtle yet so certain that it shook my worldview. In retrospect, that moment matters not because of the color I saw but because it marked the instant theory became lived experience.

You have similar anchor points—times you first felt a tingling in your palms while running them over another person's back, or that day during meditation when you saw swirls of violet behind your closed eyelids. Write them down if you have not done so. They will remind you that aura work is real, tangible, and already part of you. A personal practice grows from real moments, not from abstract aspiration. By harvesting the memories of your own discoveries, you lay down roots that will feed the routines you are about to create.

Establishing Your Core Intention

A sustainable aura healing practice begins with a clear why. Without a guiding intention you may bounce from smudging to crystal layouts to breathing exercises, feeling busy but not deeply changed. Your intention can be simple. At one stage in my life, it was "I want to feel safe in my own energy." Later it matured into "I want my presence to be a blessing for everyone I meet." Notice how each intention contains a direction—toward inner stability, toward outward service. Reflect on what feels alive in you today. Perhaps you seek relief from chronic fatigue, or maybe you want to heighten your intuition for creative work. Name it in plain language. Let it be honest rather than lofty. This single sentence becomes the compass that aligns every technique you choose.

Taking Inventory of Your Current Energy Landscape

Next comes an energetic self-assessment. Sit quietly and scan each layer of your aura as best you can, beginning near the skin and moving outward. Note the textures you perceive—dense, fluid, prickly, spacious. Where does the energy flow freely? Where does it feel sluggish or torn? You are not judging or fixing anything yet; you are simply mapping terrain. When I first performed this exercise I discovered a patch of dull gray near my left hip that pulsed with irritation any time I focused on it. Over weeks, I learned it correlated with unspoken resentment I carried from a past relationship. The mapping alone initiated healing because it revealed a truth my mind had ignored.

Pair this internal scan with practical observations of your daily life. Track your sleep quality, emotional fluctuations, and physical symptoms for at least a week. Patterns will emerge. Maybe your solar plexus tightens after long meetings, or your heart expands when you sing. These data points become the raw material from which you will craft a tailored routine.

Choosing Foundational Pillars

A house stands best on a few strong pillars, not on a cluttered web of flimsy beams. In aura healing I have found three pillars indispensable: cleansing, charging, and protecting. Cleansing removes stagnant or foreign energy. Charging infuses fresh vitality. Protecting maintains integrity in a world of mixed vibrations. Identify one method you genuinely enjoy for each pillar. Enjoyment fuels consistency. If you cringe at the smell of sage smoke, smudging will never anchor you. You might prefer a brisk salt-water shower or an imagined waterfall of gold light. For charging, maybe you love lying in sunlight or chanting vowel sounds that vibrate through your bones. For protection, you could visualize a sphere of crystalline light or wear a hematite bracelet that grounds your field. When these three practices feel natural, you have a sturdy framework onto which other techniques may be added or removed as your life evolves.

Designing a Daily Rhythm

Let us translate pillars into time. A rhythm is not a strict schedule; it is a sequence that follows the arc of your day. Morning is ideal for charging because your aura is fresh from sleep but still porous. I like to stand barefoot on the porch, breathe deeply, imagine drawing first-light energy up through my soles, and exhale it through my crown until I sense a bright halo forming. The midafternoon slump is prime for cleansing. I close my eyes at my desk, swipe my hands down my body without touching the skin, and fling any collected debris into an imaginary violet flame beside me. Evening lends itself to protection. Before bed I picture a cocoon of indigo light, thick as velvet, sealing any micro-tears incurred during the day. Find moments that fit your lifestyle. Maybe your morning commute on a train becomes your charging ritual; you rest your gaze on the passing sky and absorb vitality through your eyes. Let your practice ride the currents of daily life rather than battle them.

Weekly Deep-Dive Sessions

While daily micro-practices keep your field tidy, weekly sessions effect structural change. Reserve at least one chunk of uninterrupted time—an hour on Sunday afternoon, for example—to perform a holistic aura tune-up. My routine typically unfolds in four phases. First I cleanse with sound, sweeping two singing bowls from feet to head until I hear a consistent, clear tone. Then I repair, scanning for holes or tears using intuitive touch and mending them by drawing figure-eight patterns with my fingertips. Third, I nourish by laying crystals along my chakras, selecting stones whose colors match any dull areas I noted. Finally, I meditate in stillness, observing the new spaciousness around me. Over months these weekly sessions reshaped my aura, much like regular chiropractic adjustments realign the spine.

Design your own sequence. It might involve aromatic oils, breathwork, or guided visualization. The key is depth. Allow enough time for the subtle layers to reveal themselves. Think of it as visiting an energetic spa you built in your own living room, candles flickering, soft music playing, and an unspoken promise that this hour belongs only to your soul.

Seasonal Adjustments and Cycles

Our energy fields respond to larger rhythms as well—moon phases, tides, planetary transits, equinoxes, and solstices. Notice how your aura feels at full moon compared to new moon, how winter darkness compels you inward while summer sunshine expands you outward. My winter sessions focus more on gentle repair and nurturing warmth: I visualize thick amber honey draping over tears, slowly knitting them. Summer invites bolder charging practices: I walk under midday sun and imagine solar flares feeding every layer of my auric envelope.

You can align your practice with these cycles. Around the equinox, when light balances darkness, schedule a comprehensive aura assessment and recalibrate intentions. At solstice, celebrate by amplifying the strongest color present in your field, perhaps wearing clothing that matches it for a week. By dancing with the cosmos you remember that your aura is not an isolated bubble but part of a grand energetic choreography.

Listening to Inner Guidance

Technique is important, but intuition cements mastery. The more you practice aura work, the more you will sense subtle coaxings from within. Once, during a particularly stressful month, I set my alarm early for daily visualization. Each morning I tried to picture white light filling my aura, but I felt resistance in my chest, as though I were forcing the light. On the fourth morning, a spontaneous image arose: emerald vines growing from my heart, wrapping me in a living lattice. Relief flooded my body. The vines felt gentler than raw white brilliance, cooling the agitation I carried. Intuition presented a symbol my conscious mind would have never chosen.

Honor these whispers. If you plan to sound a tuning fork but feel drawn to hum instead, follow the impulse. If a color you have never studied appears behind your eyes during meditation, invite it in, ask its message. Your aura knows what it needs. The skill lies in listening, not controlling.

Tracking Progress Without Pressure

Because aura shifts are subtle, progress can be hard to quantify. Yet the mind craves evidence. Create a private journal exclusively for your energy journey. Record the date, techniques used, colors perceived, bodily sensations, emotional states, and any physical markers such as improved sleep or decreased headaches. Avoid evaluation language like good or bad; focus on observation: "Felt buzzing in palms, saw pale green around shoulders, mood light afterward." Over months, patterns will appear that confirm growth. Perhaps the buzzing becomes steadier, the pale green deepens to vibrant emerald, or your baseline mood elevates.

Do not let the journal become a taskmaster. If you miss entries, return without guilt. You are cultivating intimacy with yourself, not compiling a database for public review. The very act of writing slows the mind and anchors ephemeral experiences into memory, reinforcing your commitment.

Navigating Plateaus and Setbacks

Every healing path includes stagnant periods and unexpected setbacks. Sometimes life events slam into our aura like a gale, ripping newly mended tissue. Other times nothing dramatic happens; we simply stop feeling progress and wonder if the magic has evaporated. I hit one such plateau after six years of steady practice. Colors that once danced before my eyes dimmed. My weekly sessions felt routine. I considered abandoning aura work entirely. Then a friend suggested I study a new modality—Thai sound massage. The fresh perspective jolted me back into wonder, and my aura brightened again.

If you encounter a plateau, first approach with curiosity rather than judgment. Ask whether you need rest, variation, or professional support. Sometimes a two-week sabbatical from all techniques allows integration. Other times introducing a new tool—say, light language chants or flower essences—reinvigorates your field. Remember, a practice is a living organism. It sheds, renews, and sometimes cocoon in stillness before its next metamorphosis.

Creating a Sacred Physical Environment

Your aura extends beyond your skin, merging with the spaces you inhabit. Thus your home environment either supports or hinders your practice. I used to perform energy work in a cluttered apartment. Bills piled on the coffee table, half-finished crafts littered the floor. My sessions felt heavy. Eventually I dedicated a corner to aura work, cleared everything unrelated, placed a low chair, a small shelf for crystals, and a woven rug. The moment I entered that nook, my energy shifted. It signaled seriousness to my subconscious and respect to the unseen realms.

You need not carve out an entire room; a window seat or bedside table can serve. The key is consistency and intentionality. Choose colors that soothe you, instrumental music that lifts you, and lighting that mimics natural glow. Keep the space tidy and refresh it periodically with incense or flowers. When your outer environment reflects energetic harmony, your aura entrains to that vibration effortlessly.

Integrating Aura Work with Physical Practices

Because aura and body form a continuum, pairing energy work with physical disciplines multiplies results. Yoga asanas open channels, tai chi circulates qi, dance liberates stuck emotions. I often begin with ten minutes of free-form movement before settling into still aura repair; the physical motion disperses superficial static so deeper layers become accessible. Likewise, ending a session with gentle stretching grounds the newly refined energy into muscles and bones, preventing that dizzy airy feeling that sometimes follows intense spiritual work.

Diet also matters. Fresh fruits, leafy greens, and pure water supply the bio-electricity that feeds your aura. Heavy, processed foods dull it. I once kept a log correlating diet and auric perception. On days

I consumed heavy dairy and sugar, my ability to see colors faded. After three days of clean eating, clarity returned. This is not dogma but personal data. Experiment and notice your own cause-and-effect chain. The best practice is the one that honors your unique biology.

Engaging Community and Receiving Feedback

Though aura work is deeply personal, community accelerates growth. In group settings, energy fields synchronize, amplifying perceptual abilities. I learned to refine my sensing skills by exchanging readings with classmates in a weekend workshop. When five people described similar tears near my right shoulder, I could no longer dismiss that area as imagination. Their feedback compelled me to address it, which relieved chronic tension I had carried for years.

Seek trustworthy circles: meditation groups, energy-healing classes, online forums with experienced moderators. Share your observations and invite constructive insights. Community also provides accountability; knowing you will report your weekly practice encourages you to follow through. Just remember that your inner authority remains paramount. If another's interpretation feels off, thank them and return to your own knowing.

When to Consult a Professional Healer

Self-practice has limits. Serious trauma, overwhelming psychic intrusion, or complex illnesses sometimes require professional intervention. I once attempted to clear a client's energy cord attached to an abusive ex-partner. Despite my training, the cord re-established itself within hours. We eventually sought a seasoned shamanic practitioner who uncovered past-life contracts sustaining the bond. After ceremony, the cord dissolved for good.

Listen for signs you need outside help: persistent exhaustion despite regular cleansing, recurring aura holes in the same spot, or psychic phenomena beyond your skillset. Seeking assistance is not failure; it is wise stewardship of your energy field. A skilled healer can model advanced techniques you might later integrate into your own routine.

Expanding into Service

As your personal practice solidifies, you may feel called to share aura healing with others. Begin informally. Offer a short cleansing session to a friend who feels drained. Guide a family member through a protective visualization before a stressful event. Service refines your abilities. Each time you tune into another's field, you learn broader energetic languages, witness variations, and develop compassion. However, maintain boundaries. Performing healing when you are depleted degrades both auras. Uphold your pillars—cleanse, charge, protect—before and after each exchange. If the call to service deepens, consider formal training and ethical guidelines for professional practice.

Sustaining Momentum Over a Lifetime

The essence of a lifelong aura practice is adaptability. You will cycle through roles—student, explorer, teacher, beginner again. Marriage, parenthood, career changes, aging bodies—all these shifts influence your energy needs. In my thirties, rambunctious breathwork thrilled me. In my fifties, gentle humming delights me more. Permit evolution. Your aura mirrors your story, unfolding new colors, shapes, and frequencies each decade.

Schedule annual retreats, even brief ones, to review and refresh your practice. During such retreats, revisit your core intention. Perhaps it no longer resonates; craft a new statement. Try a technique you have never attempted, like biofield tuning or light grid activation. Release any practice that feels rote. Celebrate milestones: the first time you sensed your causal body, the day you saw a rainbow aura around a child. Recognize that your dedication contributes not only to your wellbeing but to the collective field of humanity, each healed aura brightening the planetary matrix.

Conclusion: Embodying the Living Light

As we close this chapter and this book, I invite you to stand wherever you are—kitchen, park bench, bedside—and feel into the space an arm's length around your body. This is your aura, a living garment of light, woven from experience, thought, emotion, and spirit. It has guided you through joys and sorrows, whispered truths in dreams, shielded you from harm, and amplified your brightest gifts. Now you have the knowledge and tools to care for it consciously and consistently.

Developing a personal aura healing practice is not about achieving perfection. It is about entering an ongoing conversation with the invisible dimension that shapes your visible life. Some days that conversation will be poetic, other days mundane. Show up anyway. Breathe, sense, and choose one small act of tending. Over time, those acts accumulate into a luminous habit, a signature frequency uniquely yours, recognizable to every soul you meet.

I began my journey awestruck by a pale blue shimmer in a grocery store. Today, decades later, my aura shines stronger because I nurtured it day after day, moment by moment. May you nurture yours with the same devotion. May your energy field grow clear and bright, resilient and kind, a beacon that lights your path and the paths of everyone fortunate enough to stand in your glow.

We began by looking at what an energy field actually is. You and I walked through the science, the spirituality, and the simple fact that every living thing glows in its own way. From there we mapped the layers of the aura, linked them to the chakras, and decoded the language of color. By the time we finished that first stretch, you knew why a murky green feels different from a bright gold.

Next, I encouraged you to get your hands dirty—or, more accurately, your eyes and your skin—by learning to see, sense, and feel those colors for yourself. We talked about the bumps and bruises an aura can collect from stress, illness, or a rough childhood. Remember the day I described my own gray haze after a month of overwork? Many readers wrote me later to say they could suddenly spot their own.

With the damage diagnosed, we opened the toolbox. You practiced smudging, sound baths, crystal grids, color breathing, and simple breathwork that costs nothing but attention. You learned how to sew up tears, sweep out sludge, and lock in fresh light with shields that flex instead of crack. Each exercise was there for you to test, tweak, and keep only if it felt right—because real healing never comes in one-size-fits-all.

Then we zoomed out. We studied the push-and-pull of relationships, how a friend's anxiety can cling like static, and how a loving hug can knit your field back together. We redesigned living rooms, work cubicles, and even phone screens to support calm energy. And the case studies—Emma's return from burnout, Luis's post-surgery recovery, my own shift from constant fatigue to steady glow—proved that steady practice beats lucky breaks every time.

So here we are at the edge of the page, but not the work. Your aura will keep changing, just as you do, and that is the best news I can give you. Meet it with curiosity, kindness, and the tools you now carry. Every breath is a chance to brighten, and every choice is another stitch in the fabric of your energy field. I will be cheering for you, light to light.

Printed in Dunstable, United Kingdom